The Impact of Pre-Transplant Red Blood Cell Transfusions in Renal Allograft Rejection

Technology Assessment Report

Project ID: RENT0610

March 7, 2012

University of Connecticut/Hartford Hospital EPC

Wendy Chen, Pharm.D., Soyon Lee, Pharm.D., Jennifer Colby, Pharm.D., Jeffrey Kluger, MD, FCC, Ajibade Ashaye, MBBS, MPH, Vanita Tongbram, MBBS, MPH, Erica Baker, Pharm.D., Jeffrey Mather, MS, Craig I Coleman, Pharm.D., C. Michael White, Pharm.D., FCP, FCCP

This report is based on research conducted by the University of Connecticut/Hartford Hospital EPC under contract to the Agency for Healthcare Research and Quality (AHRQ), Rockville, MD (RENT0610). The findings and conclusions in this document are those of the authors who are responsible for its contents. The findings and conclusions do not necessarily represent the views of AHRQ. Therefore, no statement in this report should be construed as an official position of the Agency for Healthcare Research and Quality or of the U.S. Department of Health and Human Services.

The information in this report is intended to help health care decision-makers; patients and clinicians, health system leaders, and policymakers, make well-informed decisions and thereby improve the quality of health care services. This report is not intended to be a substitute for the application of clinical judgment. Decisions concerning the provision of clinical care should consider this report in the same way as any medical reference and in conjunction with all other pertinent information, i.e., in the context of available resources and circumstances presented by individual patients.

This report may be used, in whole or in part, as the basis for development of clinical practice guidelines and other quality enhancement tools, or as a basis for reimbursement and coverage policies. AHRQ or U.S. Department of Health and Human Services endorsement of such derivative products may not be stated or implied.

None of the investigators has any affiliations or financial involvement related to the material presented in this report.

Peer Reviewers

We wish to acknowledge individuals listed below for their review of this report. This report has been reviewed in draft form by individuals chosen for their expertise and diverse perspectives. The purpose of the review was to provide candid, objective, and critical comments for consideration by the EPC in preparation of the final report. Synthesis of the scientific literature presented here does not necessarily represent the views of individual reviewers.

Maria Francesca Egidi, MD
Professor of Medicine
Medical University of South Carolina
Charleston, SC

Fred Sanfilippo, MD, PhD
Director, Healthcare Innovation Program; Professor of Pathology & Laboratory Medicine, Health Policy & Management, and Business Administration
Emory University
Atlanta, GA

Dorry Segev, MD, PhD
Associate Professor of Surgery and Epidemiology
Johns Hopkins University
Baltimore, MD

Alan Wilkinson, MD, FRCP
Professor of Medicine, Director Kidney and Pancreas Transplantation
David Geffen School of Medicine at UCLA
Los Angeles, California

Contents

Executive Summary ES-1
Background 1
    End Stage Renal Disease and Kidney Transplantation 1
    Autorecognition 1
    Allorecognition 2
    Allograft Rejection 2
        Hyperacute Rejection 2
        Acute Rejection 2
        Humoral Rejection 3
        Chronic Rejection 3
    Immunosuppression Therapy in Renal Allografts 3
        Induction Therapy 3
        Maintenance Therapy 3
    Evolution of Transfusion in Renal Transplantation 3
    Key Questions 4
        Key Question 1 4
        Key Question 2 4
Methods 6
    Literature Search Strategy 6
    Study Eligibility Criteria 6
    Data Abstraction 6
    Validity Assessment 7
    Data Synthesis 7
    Grading the Body of Evidence for Each Key Question 8
        Risk of bias 9
        Consistency 9
        Directness 9
        Precision 9
Results 10
    Study Identification and Characteristics 10
    Evaluation of Good Quality Studies 10
    Key Question 1a. Do red blood cell transfusions prior to renal transplant impact allograft rejection/survival and what is the magnitude of that effect relative to other factors (e.g., pregnancy, prior transplantation?) 14
        Univariate Analysis Results 14
        Rejection 14
        Graft Survival 14
        Patient Survival 15
        Multivariate Analysis Results 15
        Evaluation of Different Types of Transfusions on Renal Allograft Outcomes 24
    Key Question 1bi. Is any such impact of red blood cell transfusions on renal transplant outcomes altered by planned DST versus therapeutic transfusions? 27
        Univariate Analysis Results 27
        Rejection 27

- Graft Survival 28
- Patient Survival 28
- Multivariate Analysis Results 28

Key Question 1bii. Is any such impact of red blood cell transfusions on renal transplant outcomes altered by the number of transfusions, the number of units of blood, and/or the number of donors? 30
- Univariate Analysis Results 30
- Rejection 31
- Graft Survival 32
- Patient Survival 34
- Multivariate Analysis Results 35

Key Question 1biii. Is any such impact of red blood cell transfusions on renal transplant outcomes altered by the use of leukocyte-depleted blood? 43
- Rejection 44
- Graft Survival 44
- Patient Survival 44
- Rejection 47
- Graft Survival 48
- Patient Survival 48
- Panel Reactive Antibody Testing 54
- Calculated PRA Testing 55
- Impact of Sensitization on Eligibility for Transplantation 57

Key Question 2b. How useful are PRA assays in predicting sensitization from blood transfusions, donor specific antigen (DSA) sensitization, and renal transplant rejection/survival—especially in the setting of Q2a? 62
- Univariate Analysis Results 62
- Rejection 62
- Graft Survival 62
- Patient Survival 62
- Multivariate Analysis Results 63

Discussion 70
- Future Research Directions 73

Conclusion 74

References 82

Tables

Table 1. Incidence and prevalence of ESRD in patients covered by CMS by age category in 2006. 1
Table 2. Therapeutic modalities for patients with ESRD covered by CMS in 2006. 1
Table 3. Summary ratings of quality of individual studies 7
Table 4. Definitions for grading the strength of evidence..9
Table 5. Results of good quality studies on rejection 11
Table 6. Results of good quality studies on graft survival 12
Table 7. Results of good quality studies on patient survival 12
Table 8. Insight into body of literature: Transfusion versus no transfusion (KQ 1a)...............16
Table 9. Impact of transfusions (any type) on rejection (KQ 1a)...16
Table 10. Impact of transfusions (any type) on graft and patient survival (KQ1a)..................18
Table 11. Multivariate results: the impact of transfusions on rejection (KQ 1a) 19
Table 12. Multivariate results: the impact of transfusions on graft survival (KQ1a) 20
Table 13. Multivariate results: the impact of transfusions on patient survival (KQ1a)...........22
Table 14. Insight into body of literature: therapeutic/protocol transfusions versus no transfusion (excluding DST analyses) (KQ 1a)..24
Table 15. Impact of therapeutic/protocol transfusions (excluding DST analyses) on rejection (KQ 1a)...25
Table 16. Impact of therapeutic/protocol transfusion (excluding DST analyses) on graft and patient survival (KQ1a)...25
Table 17. Insight into body of literature: DST versus no transfusion (KQ 1a)........................26
Table 18. Impact of DST on rejection (KQ 1a)..26
Table 19. Impact of DST on graft and patient survival (KQ1a)...27
Table 20. Insight into body of literature: Donor-specific transfusion (KQ 1bi)......................29
Table 21. Impact of donor specific transfusion on rejection (KQ1bi) 29
Table 22. Impact of DST on graft and patient survival (KQ 1bi)..29
Table 23. Multivariate results: Impact of DST on rejection (KQ1bi)......................................30
Table 24. Multivariate results: Impact of DST on graft survival (KQ bi) 30
Table 25. Insight into body of literature: Number/Units of transfusions and number of donors (KQ1bii) 36
Table 26. Impact of any number/unit of transfusions, or number of donors on rejection (KQ1bii) 36
Table 27. Impact of number of transfusions on graft survival: intensity of transfusion versus no transfusion (KQ1bii) 37
Table 28. Impact of number of transfusions on graft survival: higher versus lower number of transfusions (KQ1bii)...37
Table 29. Impact of units of blood on graft survival: increasing number of units versus no transfusion (KQ1bii) 38
Table 30. Impact of units of blood on graft survival: greater number of units versus lower numbers of units (KQ1bii)..38
Table 31. Impact of number of transfusions on patient survival: intensity of transfusion versus no transfusion (KQ1bii) 39
Table 32. Impact of number of transfusions on patient survival: higher versus lower number of transfusions (KQ1bii)...40

Table 33. Multivariate results: Impact of number/units of transfusion on rejection (KQ1bii) 40
Table 34. Multivariate results: Impact of number/units of transfusion on graft survival (KQ1bii) 41
Table 35. Multivariate results: Impact of number/units of transfusion on patient survival (KQ1bii) 43
Table 36. Insight into body of literature: Leukocyte-depleted blood (KQ 1biii) 45
Table 37. Impact of leukocyte-depleted transfusions versus no or therapeutic transfusion on rejection (KQ 1biii) 46
Table 38. Impact of leukocyte-depleted transfusions versus no transfusion on graft and patient survival (KQ 1biii) 46
Table 39. Impact of leukocyte-depleted transfusions versus therapeutic transfusions on graft and patient survival (KQ 1biii) 46
Table 40. Insight into body of literature: Impact of transfusions over different time periods (KQ 1biv-v) 50
Table 41. Impact of transfusion over different time periods on rejection (KQ1biv-v) 51
Table 42. Impact of transfusions over different time periods on graft and patient survival (KQ 1biv-v) 52
Table 43. The impact of sensitization on the eligibility for transplantation in transfused patients 58
Table 44. Evidence depicting the association between PRA assays in predicting rejection (KQ 2b) 64
Table 45. Evidence depicting the association between PRA assays in predicting graft survival (KQ 2b)...64
Table 46. Evidence depicting the association between PRA assays in predicting patient survival (KQ 2b) 68
Table 47. Multivariate results depicting the association between PRA assays in predicting renal transplant outcomes (KQ 2b)..68
Table 48. Overview of Study Outcomes 75

Figures

Figure 1. PRISMA Diagram 13

Appendixes

Appendix A. Ovid MEDLINE Search Strategy
Appendix B. Embase Search Strategy
Appendix C. Demographics Table
Appendix D. Strength of Evidence Tables
Appendix E. Sensitization Tables

Executive Summary

Background

Over 450,000 patients in the United States have end stage renal disease (ESRD).[1] There are important morbidity and survival advantages to receiving renal transplantation versus dialysis.[2]

Human leukocyte antigens (HLA) are a set of human major histocompatibility complex derived glycoproteins that are expressed on cell surfaces and allow for discrimination of self from non-self.[1] HLA have been classified into two major groups, Class I (HLA-A, HLA-B, and HLA-C) and Class II (HLA-DP, HLA-DQ, and HLA-DR). Recognition of the antigens displayed by the transplanted organ (alloantigen) is the prime event initiating the immune response against an allograft.[1]

Hyperacute rejection is an immediate recipient immune response against an allograft due to preformed recipient antibodies directed against the donor's HLA.[1] Acute rejection is a cell mediated process that generally occurs within 5 to 90 days after a transplant, although it can rarely occur after this time. Outside of the hyperacute rejection state, humoral rejection can still occur although less frequently than cell mediated acute rejection.[3] Humoral rejection is characterized by B lymphocytes injuring the allograft through immunoglobulin and complement activities.[1] The definition of chronic rejection is ambiguous, and is sometimes recognized as chronic allograft nephropathy or any immunological responses that results in slow loss of graft function with histopathological processes: tubular atrophy, interstitial fibrosis, and fibrous intimal thickening of arteries.[4]

There have been major advances in immunosuppressive therapy.[1] Immunosuppressive therapy is broken into three categories: induction therapy, maintenance therapy, and treatment of acute rejection episodes.[1] A major advance was the use of cyclosporine and newer immunosuppressants occur in the mid 1980s and early 1990s.

High-volume use of blood transfusion was originally used in attempts to maintain ESRD patients who were anemic with red cell mass ranges of 20-25 percent. Due to concerns with transfusion-induced infections such as hepatitis and the production of anti-HLA antibodies resulting from the exposure to blood products, efforts were made in the 1970s to avoid the use of blood transfusions in renal transplant recipients.[3] During the pre-cyclosporine era, studies suggested that non-transfused renal graft recipients were at higher risk for graft rejection as compared to those transfused recipients.[5,6] Subsequently, many studies attempted to define the optimal dose and timing for the transfusion effect. With the introduction of cyclosporine in the early 1980s, leading to improved renal graft and patient survival, the beneficial role of blood transfusions and HLA matching was again being questioned. Meanwhile, some preliminary trials had shown the use of matched pretransplant blood transfusion or donor-specific transfusion (DST) to be beneficial. The evidence supporting the effects (positive, negative, neutral) of pretransplant blood transfusion, regardless of therapeutic or protocol transfusion, in renal transplantation is still not well-established. It is unclear whether the benefits, if any, of pretransplant blood transfusion may be due to the modulation of immune response in which tolerance is induced.

Objectives

This Technology Assessment evaluated data on the impact of red blood cell transfusions on renal allograft outcomes. There were two key questions with several subparts.

Key Question 1:

1a) Do red blood cell transfusions prior to renal transplant impact allograft rejection/survival and what is the magnitude of that effect relative to other factors (e.g., pregnancy, prior transplantation?)

1b) Is any such impact of red blood cell transfusions on renal transplant outcomes altered by variables such as:
  i. planned DST vs. therapeutic transfusions
  ii. the number of transfusions, the number of units of blood, and/or the number of donors
  iii. the use of leukocyte depleted blood
  iv. changes in immune-suppression regimens (pre-cyclosporine, cyclosporine, later multi-drug regimens)
  v. other changes in management over time

Key Question 2:

2a) How have panel reactive antibody (PRA) assays changed over time? Do all PRA assays measure the same things? What things contribute to intra-assay variability (e.g., time, when during the dialysis cycle the sample was obtained, statin use)? How correlative or independent of one another are these measures?

2b) How useful are PRA assays in predicting sensitization from blood transfusions, donor specific antigen (DSA) sensitization, and renal transplant rejection/survival—especially in the setting of Q2a?

Methods

Data Sources and Selection:

A systematic literature search of Medline and the Cochrane CENTRAL (from the earliest possible date through August 2010) was conducted by two independent investigators. A search of Embase (from the earliest possible date through August 2010) was conducted to identify any additional articles that were published in non-English languages. A manual review of references from pertinent articles or review articles (backward citation tracking) was conducted to identify additional articles. No language restrictions were imposed during the literature identification stage.

Titles and/or abstracts of citations identified from our literature search were assessed for full-text review if they: (1) are controlled human studies, (2) include patients who received red blood cell transfusions prior to kidney (with or without pancreas) transplantation, and (3) report on the relationship between pretransplant blood transfusion whether done for anemia management or for immune modulation or PRA assays and any renal allograft outcomes. Outcomes of interest pertaining to key question 1 include: (1) rejection, (2) graft survival, and (3) patient survival. Since the objective of key question 2a is to provide an overview of the use of panel reactive antibody (PRA) assay in renal transplant patients, there was no outcome restriction in this section and was not systematically conducted. For key question 2b, studies in a renal transplant population with use of transfusions reporting data related to the predictability of PRA assay in assessing for renal transplant rejection/survival will be included. Results published only as abstracts or poster presentations were not included in this technology assessment.

Data Extraction and Quality Assessment:

For each included study, data were collected by two investigators independently using a standardized data abstraction tool. The following information was obtained from each study (where applicable): author identification, year of publication, source of study funding, study design characteristics, population size, study period, length of study, duration of patient followup, patient baseline characteristics (e.g., donor/recipient age, duration on dialysis, cause of renal disease, and pregnancy history), prior transplantation, type of transplant, type and number of transfusions received, reason for transfusion, and PRA levels. Endpoints included: rejection, rejection, graft survival, patient survival, and degree of sensitization.

Validity assessment was performed using the recommendations in the Methods Guide for Effectiveness and Comparative Effectiveness Reviews. The following individual criteria were assessed (where applicable): comparable study groups at baseline, detailed description of study outcomes, blinding of subjects, blinding of outcome assessors, intent-to-treat analysis, description of participant withdrawals, and potential conflicts of interest. Additionally, randomized controlled trials were evaluated for randomization technique and allocation concealment. Observational studies were assessed for sample size, participant selection method, exposure measurement method, potential design biases, and appropriate analyses to adjust for confounding. Studies were assigned an overall score of good, fair, or poor.

Data Synthesis and Analysis:

In this technology assessment, we utilized in-depth tables and figure to summarize the totality of the literature. Given severe clinical and methodological heterogeneity, the retrospective nature of virtually all studies, and the inherently poor quality of individual studies upon validity assessment, we did not pool results.

Heterogeneity came from the type of transfusion (therapeutic for anemia management or donor specific for immune modulation), different definitions of endpoints, subpopulations, and etiologies of renal failure, role of HLA-matching, living versus cadaver donor, use of perioperative transfusion, previous transplant and pregnancy, history of previous random transfusion with donor-specific transfusion (DST) trials, different time periods, and ABO blood group compatibilities. In many cases, demographics were not adequately described.

We used the methods of GRADE (Grading of Recommendations Assessment, DEvelopment) to assess the strength of evidence. This system uses four required domains – risk of bias, consistency, directness, and precision. The evidence pertaining to each key question was classified into four broad categories: (1) "high", (2) "moderate", (3) "low", or (4) "insufficient" grade.

Results

There were 1274 citations identified upon our literature search with 1198 citations remaining after duplicates were removed. After title and abstract and full text review, 271 citations remained that met inclusion and exclusion criteria. One-hundred seven of these citations were duplicate reports, had overlapping populations with other studies in the search, or were summary studies without unique data not already encompassed in the search. As such, 146 unique studies were included in this technology assessment, as were 18 supplemental studies.

A summary of the results with ratings of the strength of evidence for all key questions can be found in Table ES-1. However, we are not able to provide all of the individual analyses in the limited space within the executive summary. Please see the full report for the detailed results which is vital in fully understanding the topic area.

Table ES-1. Overview of Study Outcomes

Outcome	Total Number of Analyses	Conclusion	Strength of Evidence
KEY QUESTION 1a ENDPOINTS			
REJECTION:		Transfusion has a:	
Significant Findings	25	Beneficial to no significant effect on rejection	Low
Direction of Effect	47	Beneficial to no effect on rejection	Insufficient
1-YR GRAFT SURVIVAL:		Transfusion has a:	
Significant Findings	55	Beneficial to no significant effect on graft survival	Low
Magnitude of Effect	132	Large beneficial impact or small impact on graft survival	Low
MAX DURATION GRAFT SURVIVAL:		Transfusion has a:	
Significant Findings	65	Beneficial to no significant effect on graft survival	Low
Magnitude of Effect	146	Large beneficial impact or small impact on graft survival	Low
1-YR PATIENT SURVIVAL:		Transfusion has a:	
Significant Findings	16	Beneficial to no significant effect on patient survival	Low
Magnitude of Effect	35	Large beneficial impact or small impact on patient survival	Low
MAX DURATION PATIENT SURVIVAL:		Transfusion has a:	
SignificantFindings	18	Beneficial to no significant effect on patient survival	Low
Magnitude of Effect	41	Large beneficial impact or small impact on patient survival	Low
MULTIVARIATE ANALYSES:		The covariate has:	
Prior Transplant	22	Detrimental to no significant effect on rejection, graft survival, and patient survival	Low
Transfusion	13	Beneficial to no significant effect on rejection and graft survival	Low
Pregnancy	5	Beneficial effect on rejection but detrimental to no significant effect on graft survival	Insufficient (rejection), Low (Graft Survival)
KEY QUESTION 1b i ENDPOINTS			
REJECTION:		DST Transfusion has a:	
Significant Findings	3	Beneficial to no significant effect on rejection	Low
Direction of Effect	7	Beneficial to no effect on rejection	Insufficient
1-YR GRAFT SURVIVAL:		Transfusion has a:	
Significant Findings	4	Beneficial to no significant effect on graft survival	Low
Magnitude of Effect	16	Large beneficial impact or small impact on graft survival	Low
MAX DURATION GRAFT SURVIVAL:		Transfusion has a:	
Significant Findings	5	Beneficial to no significant effect on graft survival	Low
Magnitude of Effect	17	Large beneficial impact or small impact on graft survival	Low

Outcome	Total Number of Analyses	Conclusion	Strength of Evidence
1-YR PATIENT SURVIVAL:		Transfusion has a:	
Significant Findings	2	Non-significant effect on patient survival	Insufficient
Magnitude of Effect	4	Small impact on patient survival	Low
MAX DURATION PATIENT SURVIVAL:		Transfusion has a:	
SignificantFindings	2	Non-significant effect on patient survival	Insufficient
Magnitude of Effect	4	Small impact on patient survival	Low
MULTIVARIATE ANALYSES:		The covariate has:	
DST vs Non-DST	5	Beneficial to no significant effect on rejection or graft survival	Low
KEY QUESTION 1b ii ENDPOINTS			
REJECTION: NUMBER OF TRANSFUSIONS:		Versus a lower number of transfusions, a higher number of transfusions is:	
Significant Findings	5	Beneficial to no significant effect on rejection	Low
Direction of Effect	18	Beneficial to no effect on rejection	Insufficient
NUMBER OF UNITS TRANSFUSED:		Versus no units of blood transfused, increasing number of units:	
Significant Findings	1	Non-significant effect on rejection	Insufficient
Direction of Effect	1	No effect on rejection	Insufficient

Outcome	Total Number of Analyses	Conclusion	Strength of Evidence
1-YR GRAFT SURVIVAL: NUMBER OF TRANSFUSIONS VERSUS NO TRANSFUSION:		1-5, 5-10, or >10 transfusions versus no transfusions has a:	
Significant Findings	12	Beneficial to no significant effect on graft survival	Low
Magnitude of Effect	51	Large beneficial impact or small impact on graft survival	Low
HIGHER VERSUS LOWER NUMBER OF TRANSFUSIONS:		≥5 vs. 1-5, ≥10 vs. 1-5, ≥10 vs. ≥5 transfusions has a:	
Significant Findings	11	Beneficial to no significant effect on graft survival	Low
Magnitude of Effect	43	Large beneficial impact or small impact on graft survival	Low
NUMBER OF UNITS TRANSFUSED VERSUS NO TRANSFUSION:		1-5, 5-10, or >10 transfusions versus no transfusions has a:	
Significant Findings	11	Beneficial to no significant effect on graft survival	Low
Magnitude of Effect	21	Large beneficial impact or small impact on graft survival	Low
HIGHER VERSUS LOWER NUMBER OF UNITS TRANSFUSED:		≥5 vs. 1-5, ≥10 vs. 1-5, ≥10 vs. ≥5 transfusions has a:	
Significant Findings	6	Beneficial to no significant effect on graft survival	Low
Magnitude of Effect	12	Large beneficial impact or small impact on graft survival	Low

Outcome	Total Number of Analyses	Conclusion	Strength of Evidence
MAX DURATION GRAFT SURVIVAL:			
NUMBER OF TRANSFUSIONS VERSUS NO TRANSFUSION:		1-5, 5-10, or >10 transfusions versus no transfusions has a:	
Significant Findings	9	Beneficial to no significant effect on graft survival	Low
Magnitude of Effect	53	Large beneficial impact or small impact on graft survival	Low
HIGHER VERSUS LOWER NUMBER OF TRANSFUSIONS:		$\geq$5 vs. 1-5, $\geq$10 vs. 1-5, $\geq$10 vs. $\geq$5 transfusions has a:	
Significant Findings	10	Beneficial to no significant effect on graft survival	Low
Magnitude of Effect	47	Large beneficial impact or small impact on graft survival	Low
NUMBER OF UNITS TRANSFUSED VERSUS NO TRANSFUSION:		1-5, 5-10, or >10 transfusions versus no transfusions has a:	
Significant Findings	16	Beneficial to no significant effect on graft survival	Low
Magnitude of Effect	22	Large beneficial impact or small impact on graft survival	Low
HIGHER VERSUS LOWER NUMBER OF UNITS TRANSFUSED:		$\geq$5 vs. 1-5, $\geq$10 vs. 1-5, $\geq$10 vs. $\geq$5 transfusions has a:	
Significant Findings	12	Beneficial to no significant effect on graft survival	Low
Magnitude of Effect	16	Large beneficial impact or small impact on graft survival	Low
1-YR PATIENT SURVIVAL:			
NUMBER OF TRANSFUSIONS VERSUS NO TRANSFUSION:		1-5, 5-10, or >10 transfusions versus no transfusions has a:	
Significant Findings	8	Non-significant effect on patient survival	Low
Magnitude of Effect	8	Large beneficial impact or small impact on patient survival	Low
HIGHER VERSUS LOWER NUMBER OF TRANSFUSIONS:		$\geq$5 vs. 1-5, $\geq$10 vs. 1-5, $\geq$10 vs. $\geq$5 transfusions has a:	
Significant Findings	7	No significant effect on patient survival	Low
Magnitude of Effect	7	Small impact on patient survival	Low

Outcome	Total Number of Analyses	Conclusion	Strength of Evidence
MAX DURATION PATIENT SURVIVAL:			
NUMBER OF TRANSFUSIONS VERSUS NO TRANSFUSION:		1-5, 5-10, or >10 transfusions versus no transfusions has a:	
Significant Findings	8	Non-significant effect on patient survival	Low
Magnitude of Effect	7	Large beneficial impact or small impact on patient survival	Low
HIGHER VERSUS LOWER NUMBER OF TRANSFUSIONS:		≥5 vs. 1-5, ≥10 vs. 1-5, ≥10 vs. ≥5 transfusions has a:	
Significant Findings	7	No significant effect on patient survival	Low
Magnitude of Effect	5	Small impact on patient survival	Low
MULTIVARIATE ANALYSES:		Transfusion has a:	
Transfusion of Varying Numbers vs. No Transfusion	16	Detrimental to no significant effect on rejection or graft survival	Low
>5 transfusions vs. 1-5 transfusions	4	Versus 1-5 transfusions, >5 transfusions has a: Detrimental to neutral effect on rejection and graft survival	Low
KEY QUESTION 1b iii ENDPOINTS			
1-YR GRAFT SURVIVAL:			
LEUKOCYTE DEPLETED VS. NO TRANSFUSION		Versus no transfusion, leukocyte depleted transfusion has a:	
Magnitude of Effect	2	Large beneficial impact on graft survival	Low
LEUKOCYTE DEPLETED VS. TRANSFUSION:		Versus transfusion, leukocyte depleted transfusion has a:	
Significant Findings	1	Non-significant effect on graft survival	Insufficient
Magnitude of Effect	2	Small change in graft survival	Low
MAX DURATION GRAFT SURVIVAL:			
LEUKOCYTE DEPLETED VS. NO TRANSFUSION		Versus no transfusion, leukocyte depleted transfusion has a:	
Magnitude of Effect	2	Large beneficial impact on graft survival	Low
LEUKOCYTE DEPLETED VS. TRANSFUSION:		Versus transfusion, leukocyte depleted transfusion has a:	
Significant Findings	1	Non-significant effect on graft survival	Insufficient
Magnitude of Effect	2	Large beneficial effect or small change in graft survival	Low

Outcome	Total Number of Analyses	Conclusion	Strength of Evidence
MAX DURATION PATIENT SURVIVAL: LEUKOCYTE DEPLETED VS. NO TRANSFUSION			
Magnitude of Effect	1	No effect on rejection	Insufficient
LEUKOCYTE DEPLETED VS. TRANSFUSION:			
Significant Findings	1	No significant effect on rejection	Insufficient
Magnitude of Effect	1	No effect on rejection	Insufficient
KEY QUESTION 1b iv-v ENDPOINTS			
REJECTION:		Over progressive time periods transfusion has a:	
Significant Findings	11	Up to the year 1992, transfusion had a significant beneficial to neutral effect but after 1992, it may not have this effect	Low
Direction of Effect	35	Up to the year 1992, transfusion had a beneficial to neutral effect but after 1992, it may not have this effect	Low
1-YR GRAFT SURVIVAL:		Over progressive time periods transfusion has a:	
Significant Findings	47	Transfusion had a significant beneficial to neutral effect	Low
Magnitude of Effect	108	Transfusion has a large beneficial impact or small impact on graft survival	Low
MAX DURATION GRAFT SURVIVAL:		Over progressive time periods transfusion has a:	
Significant Findings	57	Transfusion had a significant beneficial to neutral effect	Low
Magnitude of Effect	119	Transfusion has a large beneficial impact or small impact on graft survival	Low
1-YR PATIENT SURVIVAL:		Over progressive time periods transfusion has a:	
Significant Findings	17	Transfusion had a significant beneficial to neutral effect	Low
Magnitude of Effect	30	Transfusion has a large beneficial impact or small impact on patient survival	Low
MAX DURATION PATIENT SURVIVAL:		Over progressive time periods transfusion has a:	
Significant Findings	18	Transfusion had a significant beneficial to neutral effect	Low
Magnitude of Effect	37	Transfusion has a large beneficial impact or small impact on patient survival	Low
KEY QUESTION 2b ENDPOINTS			
REJECTION:		Lower PRA% is associated with a:	
Significant Findings	2	Non-significant effect on rejection	Low
Direction of Effect	2	Directionally less rejection	Insufficient

Outcome	Total Number of Analyses	Conclusion	Strength of Evidence
1-YR GRAFT SURVIVAL:		Lower PRA% is associated with a:	
Significant Findings	8	Significant beneficial to neutral effect	Low
Direction of Effect	11	Large beneficial impact or small impact on graft survival	Low
MAX DURATION GRAFT SURVIVAL:		Lower PRA% is associated with a:	
Significant Findings	14	Significant beneficial to neutral effect on graft survival	Low
Direction of Effect	18	Large beneficial impact or small impact on graft survival	Low
MAX DURATION PATIENT SURVIVAL:		Lower PRA% is associated with a:	
Significant Findings	2	Non-significant effect on patient survival	Low
MULTIVARIATE ANALYSES:		Lower PRA is:	
Rejection	2	Not an independent predictor of lower rejection	Low
Graft Survival	7	Significant beneficial to neutral effect of graft survival	Low
Patient Survival	3	Significant beneficial to neutral effect on patient survival	Low

PRA = Panel Reactive Antibodies, YR = Year

Discussion

Although we evaluated a voluminous literature set, the studies were predominantly retrospective, did not account for confounding, and in many cases had sparse reporting of demographics. The studies also had very high clinical and methodological heterogeneity precluding the ability to pool results. This heterogeneity was due to the different definitions of endpoints of interest, differing subpopulations of patients, different etiologies of renal failure, studies with and without any HLA-matching, differing cold ischemia times, the use of or different mixture of living versus deceased donors, use of perioperative transfusion, previous transplant or pregnancy history, history of previous random transfusions in patients receiving DST, differing followup periods, and ABO blood incompatibilities. This high degree of clinical and methodological heterogeneity precluded the ability to pool the results.

We chose to evaluate our data based on the percentage of analyses evaluating an endpoint that either showed a significant effect (either beneficial or detrimental) or a non-significant effect. We then evaluated our data based on the direction and/or magnitude of effect (either beneficial or detrimental). This approach has limitations because analyses of varying quality and sample size were evaluated together but it provides that only type of independent qualitative analyses that can be done on such a literature base.

In the vast majority of analyses reporting the significance of their findings, the use of transfusions versus no transfusions either resulted in a significantly beneficial or insignificant effect on rejection, graft survival, or patient survival. When analyses were evaluated regardless of the significance of the findings, which allows underpowered analyses and analyses for which the original study authors did not discern the significance of their findings to be included, we found that the use of transfusions versus no transfusions either resulted in either beneficial or small/null effects on rejection, graft survival, or patient survival. For the analyses evaluating the impact of the use of larger number of transfusion/transfused units versus no, or a smaller number of transfusions/transfused units, we found mixed effect on rejection, graft survival or patient survival. So the literature, weak as it is, demonstrates a neutral to positive effect resulting from transfusion and does not reflect a detrimental effect resulting from transfusion. The same results were found when comparing DST with non-DST transfusions or leukocyte depleted/free transfusions with no or non-leukocyte depleted/free transfusions with either neutral or beneficial effects resulting.

In our Technology Assessment, having a lower PRA due to transfusion generally has a beneficial to neutral effect on outcomes. These data are limited because it does not consistently define PRA in the same manner (Peak or Current PRA), does not allow assessment for the specific HLA antibodies that the patients are incompatible with (like is becoming the standard of care with "calculated PRA"), the assays for PRA have inter and intra-assay variability, there are modulators of PRA level and the use of these modulators are not specified in the studies, the time course from exposure to transfusion or other stimuli to the time the PRA is recorded is not defined, and most importantly that the degree to which the elevated PRA in these studies were due to transfusions versus other stimuli such as transplants or other factors such as pregnancy cannot be determined. It should be noted that PRA is a surrogate measure for immunization, and its link to renal allograft outcomes is tenuous due to the myriad confounding factors such as donor types, immunosuppression used, and other factors that can influence the transplant outcomes. The purpose of this TA is not to identify a specific causal link between PRA and renal allograft outcomes, but rather to examine the available data to identify the correlation between the two in studies that did assess transfusion use and final health outcomes.

There are problems with internal validity and heterogeneity with these individual studies. As such, we have low confidence that the evidence reflects the true effect. Further research is likely to change our confidence in the estimate of effect and likely change the estimate as well. In addition, the findings of our Technology Assessment need to be viewed in light of one very important limitation. The studies, as devised, evaluated the impact of transfusions on transplantation outcomes but could only be determined among those patients who actually received transplantation. In several of our included studies, we found that a proportion of patients who were sensitized after transfusion ended up not being considered for their planned kidney and had a delay in transplantation, received a different organ type (deceased versus living), had to undergo a procedure to attenuate sensitization such as plasmapheresis, or went back on the waiting list. In some cases, patients reportedly died while on the waiting list. As such, we cannot be sure that transfusions have a beneficial to neutral effect on transplantation outcomes or select out those most likely to be successful after transplantation. It is unclear why intention-to-treat analyses were not utilized by investigators, where possible.

There are data from large registries that are published in non-peer reviewed book chapters, do not have an adequate description of methods, and in most cases do not account for a myriad of confounders. While they did not make our a priori criteria for study inclusion, they do provide provocative data that should be noted. There are at least six book chapters within the Clinical Transplants textbook that uses data from the UCLA or UNOS registries. In one book chapter using the UCLA Transplant Registry over a ten year period (1981 to 1990), the 1-year graft survival in patients undergoing first transplants was significantly better in unsensitized patients (PRA 0-10%) versus those with a PRA >50% in 5 of the 10 years.[7] In the same book chapter, using data from the UCLA Transplant Registry from 1985 to 1990 or the UNOS Registry from 1987 to 1990 (the source of the evidence was not specified), the authors found that receiving more transfusions increased the number of patients undergoing a first transplant becoming sensitized. Given these two pieces of indirect evidence, it would seem intuitive that transfusions would negatively impact 1-year graft survival but like the analyses that made it into our Technology Assessment, transfusions either had a beneficial or neutral effect in both males and females who had a PRA of 0-10%, PRA of 11-50%, or PRA of >50%. Clearly there is a disconnect in logic that may suggest: (1) the benefits of reducing graft rejection through a non-PRA mechanism of transfusion overcomes the negative effect of raising PRA on graft rejection; (2) transfusions self-select those with the greater ability to do well after transplantation; or (3) another confounder explains the discrepancy but has not been evaluated. It is possible that the avoidance of incompatible organs attenuates the negative impact of elevated PRA on outcomes but in so doing, decreases the available pool of organs. This is plausible since in this book chapter, the waiting time for an organ is prolonged in both males and females when PRAs are elevated. Another chapter from this textbook using UNOS data from 1995 to 2000 shows that increasing the number of transfusions qualitatively increased the number of sensitized patients and reduced graft survival, although statistical analyses were not provided.[8] In book chapter from an earlier edition of the textbook, UNOS Registry data from 1988 to 1996 was reported. It reported that increasing numbers of transfusions significantly increased sensitization (higher PRAs) and that elevated PRA (from any cause) was qualitatively associated with worse graft survival although statistical results for this latter analysis were not provided.[9] In another book chapter, UCLA Registry data from 1981 to 1990 found qualitatively better 1-year graft survival annually from 1981 through 1987, similar 1-year graft survival from 1988 to 1989, and worse survival in 1990 in those with one or more transfusions versus no transfusions although the authors suggested that the 1990 data could be a spurious result produced by late reporting of followup.[10] UNOS Registry data from 1987 to 1990 found similar 1-year graft survival in those with one or more transfusions versus no transfusions. Another book chapter using UNOS data reiterated similar risks of higher numbers of transfusions increasing risk of developing higher PRAs and higher PRAs (from any source) increasing risk of graft failure[11] while another book chapter reiterated that patients with PRAs >50% (from any cause) have longer waiting times for transplantation.[12]

In the USRDS Annual Data Report in 2010, patients with higher PRAs have longer waiting times.[13] Receiving a transfusion while on the transplant waiting list is associated with a 5-fold higher risk of dying while on the wait list within the first five years and an 11% reduction in the likelihood of receiving a transplant within the first 5-years. Why such a disparity exists between the relatively small reduction in transplantation and the large increase in the likelihood of death of the waiting list is unclear. The data was adjusted for age, gender, race, ethnicity, cause of end stage renal disease, blood type, body mass index, pretransplant time on dialysis, education, dialysis type, and comorbid conditions. It could be that while the risk of having no transplant within 5 years is low, the prolongation of waiting time leads to poorer outcomes, there is ultimately a poorer match, or transfusion may be a marker of some other underlying disorder that hastens death unrelated to the transfused product itself. Ultimately, these data did not meet our inclusion criteria and were not included in our results section. While the data provided by USRDS on overall transplant outcomes is extensive, the USRDS report was not focused on the direct impact of transfusions on transplant outcomes. The USRDS data collection system is limited to self-reporting of transfusion status in transplant candidates and recipients, in which it is limited to discrete data (i.e. yes, no, or unknown) on whether patients have received transfusions while the indications and/or appropriateness of the transfusions are often unknown. As such, the direct correlation of sensitization and transfusion cannot be established.

Future Research Directions

We believe that additional adequately powered studies should be conducted. In these studies we believe that they should be multi-institutional because individual center practices and procedures are so variable, have adequate reporting of demographics and either use statistical means to account for confounders (propensity score adjustment or matching) or use of randomization, have standard definitions of outcomes, and have a standard followup time of at least 1-year. Patients receiving or being randomized to no transfusions should be screened to assure that this not only includes transfusions within the dialysis or transplant center but other transfusions as well. We believe that standard PRA testing should be supplanted with updated CPRA testing so that specific HLA antigen sensitivities resulting from transfusions can be identified and perhaps correlated with outcomes. Outcomes such as sensitization rate, access to transplantation, and waiting time to transplantation during the pretransplant time period as well as graft outcomes during post-transplant period should be evaluated.

The impact of different immunosuppressive regimens (induction and maintenance as well as novel therapies such as statins) on outcomes in patients receiving transfusions to identify those regimens which can suppress the advantageous or detrimental effects of transfusion on outcomes is needed. This should be specifically evaluated to determine whether transfusions need to be encouraged, avoided, or matched with certain regimens. Such evaluations should adhere to good study conduction practices.

Data from large scale registries could be used for future research but should be published in peer reviewed journals, have an adequate use and description of methods, have a reliable and objective data collection system, as well as account for a myriad of confounders.

Conclusion

Transfusions generally have beneficial to neutral effects on renal allograft outcomes, and have minimal detrimental effects on the outcomes for renal transplant recipients. There is not much support for the notion that transfusions increase the risk of graft rejection among those receiving transplantation. Although there is evidence that patients receiving pretransplant transfusions have increased levels of sensitization as assessed by PRA, the relationship between the number of pretransplant transfusions and the extent of levels of sensitization is still not established. It should be noted that in some studies, patients who were candidates for transplantation were ultimately not offered the transplant due to high PRA levels. Some other studies did not disclose the number of patients who were ultimately not transplanted due to a high PRA as they focused on the population undergoing transplant. This is a major confounder in these studies.

When we examine results based on advancing time periods (before 1942, 1984-1991, and 1992 to the present), the percentage of analyses showing benefit is attenuated in more recently conducted studies. With regard to rejection, the data are more ambiguous with some analyses showing benefit, some showing a neutral effect, and other analyses showing harm, although the number of studies evaluating more recent time periods is quite limited.

In essence, the literature base is weak and future research conducted with proper control for confounders, disclosure of baseline characteristics, and use of other good study design techniques is needed to assess the impact of transfusions on allograft and patient survival outcomes in renal transplant recipients.

Glossary:

DST = Donor Specific Transfusion. Transfusions using the donor's blood.
ESRD = End Stage Renal Disease. The final and most severe stage of renal disease.
HLA = Human Leukocyte Antigen. Antigens that allow the immune system to discern self from non-self.
PRA = Panel Reactive Antibodies. A determination of the extent to which a recipient is sensitized.

References

Please refer to the reference list in the full report for documentation of statements contained in the Executive Summary.

Background

End Stage Renal Disease and Kidney Transplantation

Over 450,000 patients in the United States have end stage renal disease (ESRD).[1] While there are important morbidity and survival advantages to receiving renal transplantation versus dialysis modalities, only 14,059 kidney transplants were performed in 2009.[2] The Coverage and Analysis Group at the Centers for Medicare and Medicaid Services (CMS) requested a report from The Technology Assessment Program (TAP) at the Agency for Healthcare Research and Quality (AHRQ) that assessed the impact of renal transplantation on renal allograft endpoints. AHRQ assigned this report to the University of Connecticut/Hartford Hospital Evidence-based Practice Center (Contract Number: 290 2007 10067 I). The technology assessment focused on two key questions with several subparts.

Most patients with ESRD who require dialysis for four or more months qualify for Center for Medicare & Medicaid Services (CMS) coverage until dialysis ceases. Renal transplantation and subsequent care in patients with ESRD is also covered for three years after transplantation. The likelihood of transplantation within three years of ESRD registration is 17.8 percent but varies from 9.2 percent in those 60 to 69 years of age to 69.9 percent in those 0 to 19 years of age. (2003 United States Renal Data System) The incidence and prevalence of ESRD in patients covered by CMS by age category in 2006 is provided in Table 1. The use of hemodialysis, transplant, transplantation wait list, or peritoneal dialysis in patients covered by CMS in 2006 is provided in Table 2.

Table 1. Incidence and prevalence of ESRD in patients covered by CMS by age category in 2006.

Age	Incidence #	Incidence %	Prevalence #	Prevalence %	*Treatment Composition*
0-19	1,303	1.2	7,465	1.5	Mostly transplant
20-44	13,977	12.6	96,677	19.1	Almost equal
45-64	41,729	37.6	223,374	44.1	2:1 dialysis: transplant
65-74	25,500	23.0	99,431	19.6	Primarily dialysis
75+	28,342	25.6	79,308	15.7	Primarily dialysis
Unknown	-------	-------	-------	-------	-------

Table 2. Therapeutic modalities for patients with ESRD covered by CMS in 2006.

	New Patients 2006	Total Patients 2006
Hemodialysis	101,306	327,754
Transplant	2,635	151,502
Transplant Wait List	---------	68,576
Peritoneal Dialysis	6,725	26,082

Autorecognition

Human leukocyte antigens (HLA) are a set of human major histocompatibility complex derived glycoproteins that are expressed on cell surfaces and allow for discrimination of self from non-self.[1] HLA have been classified into two major groups, Class I (HLA-A, HLA-B, and HLA-C) and Class II (HLA-DP, HLA-DQ, and HLA-DR). Class I HLA molecules are expressed on the surface of all nucleated cells and are recognized by cytotoxic T cells (CD8+). Cytotoxic T cells promote target cell destruction through apoptosis and release of cytotoxic proteins. Class II HLA molecules are expressed solely on the surfaces of antigen- presenting cells (APCs). APCs include dendritic cells, macrophages, and activated B lymphocytes. APCs are vital in initiating the immune response and stimulating helper T cells (CD4+). Some T helper cells secrete cytokines that recruit cytotoxic T cells, B lymphocytes, or APCs while others secrete cytokines which attenuate the immune response. When a B lymphocyte binds to an antigen and receives a cytokine signal from a helper T cell, it can differentiate into a plasma B cell or a memory B cell. Plasma B cells secrete antibodies which can destroy target antigens while memory B cells cause long term immunity and rapidly activate the immune system upon subsequent exposure to the target antigen.[1]

Allorecognition

Recognition of the antigens displayed by the transplanted organ (alloantigen) is the prime event initiating the immune response against an allograft.[1] In the direct pathway, donor APCs migrate to the recipient's lymph nodes and present donor HLA glycoproteins to T cells. In the indirect pathway, recipient APCs migrate into the allograft and phagocytize alloantigens. The HLA glycoproteins are then presented to recipient T cells in the lymph nodes. Regardless of whether the alloantigen is presented via the direct or indirect pathway (referred to as *Signal 1*), a second costimulatory signal (referred to as *Signal 2*) must also take place for T cell activation. This is an interaction between one of several costimulatory receptors and paired ligands on the surfaces of APCs and T cells.[1]

Allograft Rejection

Hyperacute Rejection

Hyperacute rejection is an immediate recipient immune response against an allograft due to preformed recipient antibodies directed against the Donor's HLA.[1] Those at highest risk have HLA or ABO blood group antibodies including patients with a history of previous organ transplantation, multiple blood transfusions, and mothers receiving organs from their children.[1]

Acute Rejection

Acute rejection is a cell mediated process that generally occurs within 5 to 90 days after a transplant, although it can occur after this time.[1] Unlike the B lymphocyte mediated hyperacute rejection, this reaction is mediated through alloreactive T cells. Activated cytotoxic T cells infiltrate the graft and trigger an immune response. They can induce graft injury by inducing apoptosis and by secreting cytotoxic proteins (perforin and ganzyme B). Pretransplant assessment for the presence or absence of alloantibodies and T cell activities to HLA antigens is touted to reduce the risk of acute rejection. Clinical symptoms associated with acute rejection of a renal allograft include fever, allograft tenderness, decreased urine output, malaise, hypertension, weight gain, and edema. Clinical signs include increases in serum creatinine, blood urea nitrogen, leukocyte concentrations, allograft swelling, and a positive renal biopsy for lymphocyte infiltration.[1]

Humoral Rejection

Outside of the hyperacute rejection state, humoral rejection can still occur although less frequently than cell mediated acute rejection.[3] Humoral rejection is characterized by B lymphocytes injuring the allograft through immunoglobulin and complement activities.[1]

Chronic Rejection

The definition of chronic rejection is ambiguous, and is sometimes recognized as chronic allograft nephropathy or any immunological responses that results in slow loss of graft function with histopathological processes: tubular atrophy, interstitial fibrosis, and fibrous intimal thickening of arteries.[4]

Immunosuppression Therapy in Renal Allografts

There have been major advances in immunosuppressive therapy.[1] Immunosuppressive therapy is broken into three categories: induction therapy, maintenance therapy, and treatment of acute rejection episodes.[1]

Induction Therapy

Induction therapy is usually initiated intraoperatively or immediately after the transplant and continues for 7 to 10 days.[1] Induction agents include basiliximab, daclizumab, antithymocyte globulin equine, antithymocyte globulin rabbit, and muromonab-CD3, and alemtuzumab. Induction therapy is not a uniformly used but is often considered for those with preformed antibodies, history of previous organ transplantation, multiple HLA mismatches, or transplantation of organs with prolonged cold ischemic time, or from expanded criteria donors. These therapies are not without the potential for harms resulting from opportunistic infections and malignancy.[1]

Maintenance Therapy

Maintenance therapy is routinely provided to patients and available classes include: calcineurin inhibitors (cyclosporine and tacrolimus), antiproliferatives (azathioprine and mycophenylate acid derivatives), target of Rapamycin inhibitors (sirolimus) and corticosteroids (prednisolone and dexamethasone).[1] Maintenance therapy is generally achieved by selecting two or more medications from different classes to maximize efficacy while minimizing adverse effects.[1]

Evolution of Transfusion in Renal Transplantation

High-volume therapeutic use of blood transfusion was originally used in attempts to maintain ESRD patients who were anemic with red cell mass ranges of 20-25 percent. Due to concerns with transfusion-induced infections such as hepatitis and the production of anti-HLA antibodies resulting from the exposure to blood products, efforts were made in the 1970s to avoid the use of blood transfusions in renal transplant recipients.[3] During the pre-cyclosporine era, studies suggested that non-transfused renal graft recipients were at higher risk for graft rejection as compared to those transfused recipients.[5,6] Subsequently, many studies attempted to define the optimal dose and timing for the transfusion effect. With the introduction of cyclosporine in the early 1980s, leading to improved renal graft and patient survival, the beneficial role of blood transfusions and HLA matching was again being questioned. Meanwhile, some preliminary trials had shown the use of per-protocol transfusion: matched pretransplant blood transfusion (mPTFs) or donor-specific transfusion (DST) to be beneficial. The evidence supporting the effects (positive, negative, neutral) of pretransplant blood transfusion, regardless of therapeutic or protocol transfusion, in renal transplantation is still not well-established. It is unclear whether the benefits, if any, of pretransplant blood transfusion may be due to the modulation of immune response in which tolerance is induced.

Key Questions

The following key questions were formulated to evaluate current literature on the impact of pre-transplant red blood cell transfusion in renal allograft outcomes:

Key Question 1:

1a) Do red blood cell transfusions prior to renal transplant impact allograft rejection/survival and what is the magnitude of that effect relative to other factors (e.g., pregnancy, prior transplantation?)

1b) Is any such impact of red blood cell transfusions on renal transplant outcomes altered by variables such as:
   i. planned DST vs. therapeutic transfusions
   ii. the number of transfusions, the number of units of blood, and/or the number of donors
   iii. the use of leukocyte depleted blood
   iv. changes in immune-suppression regimens (pre-cyclosporine, cyclosporine, later multi-drug regimens)
   v. other changes in management over time

Key Question 2:

2a) How have panel reactive antibody (PRA) assays changed over time? Do all PRA assays measure the same things? What things contribute to intra-assay variability (e.g., time, when during the dialysis cycle the sample was obtained, statin use)? How correlative or independent of one another are these measures?

2b) How useful are PRA assays in predicting sensitization from blood transfusions, donor specific antigen (DSA) sensitization, and renal transplant rejection/survival—especially in the setting of Q2a?

Methods

Literature Search Strategy

A systematic literature search of Medline and the Cochrane CENTRAL (from the earliest possible date through August 2010) was conducted by two independent investigators. A search of Embase (from the earliest possible date through August 2010) was conducted to identify any additional articles that were published in non-English languages. A manual review of references from pertinent articles or review articles (backward citation tracking) was conducted to identify additional articles. No language restrictions were imposed during the literature identification stage. The search strategy was designed to answer both key questions 1 and 2, and is available in Appendix A.

Study Eligibility Criteria

Two investigators independently determined study eligibility, with disagreements resolved by discussion or by a third investigator. Titles and/or abstracts of citations identified from our literature search were assessed for full-text review if they: (1) were controlled human studies, (2) included patients who received red blood cell transfusions prior to kidney (with or without pancreas) transplantation, and (3) reported on the relationship between pretransplant blood transfusion whether done for anemia management or for immune modulation or PRA assays and any renal allograft outcomes. Outcomes of interest pertaining to key question 1 include: (1) rejection, (2) graft survival, and (3) patient survival. Since the objective of key question 2a was to provide an overview of the use of panel reactive antibody (PRA) assay in renal transplant patients, there are no outcome restrictions in this section and were not systematically conducted. For key question 2b, studies reporting data related to the predictability of PRA assay in assessing the sensitization from blood transfusions, donor specific antigen sensitization, and renal transplant rejection/survival were included. Results published only as abstracts or poster presentations were not included in this technology assessment.

Data Abstraction

For each included study, data were collected by two investigators independently using a standardized data abstraction tool. The following information was obtained from each study (where applicable): author identification, year of publication, source of study funding, study design characteristics, population size, study period, length of study, duration of patient followup, patient baseline characteristics (e.g., donor/recipient age, duration on dialysis, cause of renal disease, and pregnancy history), prior transplantation, type of transplant, type and number of transfusions received, reason for transfusion, and PRA levels. Endpoints included: rejection, graft survival, patient survival, and degree of sensitization.

Validity Assessment

Validity assessment was performed using the recommendations in the Methods Guide for Effectiveness and Comparative Effectiveness Reviews. The following individual criteria were assessed (where applicable): comparable study groups at baseline, detailed description of study outcomes, blinding of subjects, blinding of outcome assessors, intent-to-treat analysis, description of participant withdrawals, and potential conflicts of interest. Additionally, randomized controlled trials were evaluated for randomization technique and allocation concealment. Observational studies were assessed for sample size, participant selection method, exposure measurement method, potential design biases, and appropriate analyses to adjust for confounding. Studies were assigned an overall score of good, fair, or poor (Table 3). This rating system does not attempt to assess the comparative validity across different types of study design. For example, a "fair" randomized controlled trial should not be implied to have the same methodological criteria as a "fair" observational study. Both study design and quality rating should be considered when interpreting the methodological quality of a study.

Table 3. Summary ratings of quality of individual studies

Quality Rating	Definition
Good (low risk of bias)	These studies have the least bias and results are considered valid. A study that adheres mostly to the commonly held concepts of high quality include the following: a formal randomized, controlled study; clear description of the population, setting, interventions, and comparison groups; appropriate measurement of outcomes; appropriate statistical and analytic methods and reporting; no reporting errors; less than 20 percent dropout; and clear reporting of dropouts.
Fair	These studies are susceptible to some bias, but it is not sufficient to invalidate results. They do not meet all the criteria required for a rating of good quality because they have some deficiencies, but no flaw is likely to cause major bias. The study may be missing information, making it difficult to assess limitations and potential problems.
Poor (high risk of bias)	These studies have significant flaws that imply biases of various types that may invalidate the results. They have serious errors in design, analysis, or reporting; large amounts of missing information, or discrepancies in reporting.

Data Synthesis

In this technology assessment, we utilized in-depth tables and figure to summarize the totality of the literature. Given severe clinical and methodological heterogeneity, the retrospective nature of virtually all studies, and the inherently poor quality of individual studies upon validity assessment, we did not pool results.

Heterogeneity came from the type of transfusion (therapeutic for anemia management or donor specific for immune modulation), different definitions of endpoints, subpopulations, and etiologies of renal failure, role of HLA-matching, living versus cadaver donor, use of perioperative transfusion, previous transplant and pregnancy, history of previous random transfusion with donor-specific transfusion (DST) trials, different time periods, and ABO blood group compatibilities. In many cases, demographics were not adequately described.

Grading the Body of Evidence for Each Key Question

We used the criteria and methods of GRADE (Grading of Recommendations Assessment, DEvelopment) to assess the strength of evidence. This system uses four required domains – risk of bias, consistency, directness, and precision. All assessments were made by two investigators (with disagreements resolved through discussion). The evidence pertaining to each key question was classified into four broad categories: (1) "high", (2) "moderate", (3) "low", or (4) "insufficient" grade. Below we describe in more detail the features that determined the strength of evidence for the different outcomes evaluated in this report (Table 4).

Table 4. Definitions for grading the strength of evidence

Grade	Definition
High	There is high confidence that the evidence reflects the true effect. Further research is very unlikely to change our confidence in the estimate of effect.
Moderate	Moderate confidence that the evidence reflects the true effect. Further research may change our confidence in the estimate of effect and may change the estimate.
Low	Low confidence that the evidence reflects the true effect. Further research is likely to change our confidence in the estimate of effect and is likely to change the estimate.
Insufficient	Evidence either is unavailable or does not permit estimation of an effect

Risk of bias

Risk of bias is the degree to which the included studies, for any given outcome or comparison, have a high likelihood of adequate protection against bias. This can be assessed through the evaluation of both design and study limitations.

Consistency

Consistency refers to the degree of similarity in the direction of the effect sizes from included studies within an evidence base. This was assessed in two main ways: 1) the effect sizes had the same sign, in that they were on the same side of unity; 2) the range of effect sizes was narrow.

Directness

Directness refers to whether the evidence links the compared interventions directly with health outcomes, and compares two or more interventions in head-to-head trials. Indirectness implies that more than one body of evidence is required to link interventions to the most important health outcomes.

Precision

Precision refers to the degree of certainty surrounding effect estimate(s) with respect to a given outcome. A precise estimate is an estimate that would allow a clinically useful conclusion. An imprecise estimate is one for which the confidence interval is wide enough to include clinically distinct conclusions (e.g. both clinically important superiority and inferiority), a circumstance that will preclude a conclusion.

Results

Study Identification and Characteristics

As delineated in the PRISMA diagram (Figure 1), there were 1274 citations identified upon our literature search with 1198 citations remaining after duplicates were removed. After title and abstract and full text review, 271 citations remained that met inclusion and exclusion criteria. One-hundred seven of these citations were duplicate reports, had overlapping populations with other studies in the search, or were summary studies without unique data not already encompassed in the search. As such, 146 unique studies were included in this technology assessment, as were 18 supplemental studies.

In each section we report the number of studies and their univariate analyses that evaluated for rejection, graft survival, and patient survival. Information on the studies germane to multivariate analyses is reported in those subsections.

Key characteristics of each unique study may be found in Appendix C. Of the 146 unique studies included in this report, 119 (82 percent) were retrospective observational studies, 15 (10 percent) for prospective observational studies and 12 (8 percent) for clinical controlled trials. Over half of the studies included in this technology assessment were conducted before 1984, and fewer than ten percent of the studies were conducted after 1992. Hundred and twelve of 146 (77 percent) of the studies did not account for confounders by using statistical methods such as propensity score adjustment or randomization. Seventy-three percent of the studies did not report demographics for the population of interest for this technology assessment. Over one-third of the included studies were conducted in the United States, and fewer than one percent of the studies were multicenter studies. For the assessments of the strength of the body of evidence for each key question, see Appendix D.

Evaluation of Good Quality Studies

Of the 146 unique studies included in the evaluation of the impact of transfusion, only five studies were rated as good quality studies, all of which were clinical controlled trials.[14-18] Amongst the five good quality studies, three (60 percent) evaluated the impact of donor specific transfusion on renal allograft outcomes (i.e. rejection, graft and patient survival), while the remaining two (40 percent) evaluated protocol transfusion (therapeutic transfusion given when necessary). (Table 5–Table 7) All studies provided outcomes on graft rejection, graft and patient survival.

Nine analyses reported results on rejection frequency, defined as the percent of patients treated for rejection, patients with at least one rejection episode or rejection rate per patient. Of the five analyses reporting on the statistical significance of their results, two found significant reductions in rejection episodes in patients receiving transfusion (one for DST and the other for random transfusion), one found the use of DST significantly increased total number of rejection episodes, and the remaining two found no significant differences in transfused patients as compared to the control group. (Table 5)

Of all these good quality studies, only one study provided a definition of graft survival.[16] Two of the five studies reported the statistical significance of the results.

While one of them found that transfusion significantly improved 1-year and maximum duration of graft survival,[17] the other study found that donor-specific transfusions did not have a significant impact on 1-year graft survival (which was the maximum duration as well), although there was a trend towards improvement with the use of donor-specific transfusions.[18] The remaining three studies that did not report statistical significance of the results found that transfusions (regardless transfusion types) had a beneficial to neutral direction of effect on 1-year and maximum duration graft survival.[14-16] (Table 6).

Two of the five studies[15,17] reported three analyses in which transfusions did not have any significant effect on 1-year patient survival while one of the studies[17] found no significant impact on maximum duration patient survival as well. The other three studies found donor-specific transfusions to have a neutral effect on 1–year and maximum duration of patient survival, but the significance of the results was not reported. (Table 7)

Table 5. Results of good quality studies on rejection

Study, Year	Intervention	Graft Rejection Definition	Graft Rejection (%)	P-value
Marti HP et al, 2006	DST (n=55)	Patients treated for acute renal allograft rejection during the first year after living renal allograft transplantation	6	NR
	Control (n=55)		14	
Hiesse C et al, 2001a*	DR-matched transfusion (n=31)	Patients treated for biopsy-confirmed acute rejection episodes during the six-month post-transplant period	19	NR
	No Transfusion (n=36)		33	
Hiesse C et al, 2001b*	DR-mismatched transfusion (n=39)	Patients treated for biopsy-confirmed acute rejection episodes during the six-month post-transplant period	33	NR
	No Transfusion (n=36)		33	
Alexander JW et al, 1999 §	DST (n=115) Control (n=97)	Patients with biopsy-confirmed rejection episodes	70 56	NR
	DST (n=115) Control (n=97)	Patients reporting at least one rejection	52 45	0.32
Opelz G et al, 1997 §	Transfusion (n=205) No transfusion (n=218)	Patients not treated for rejection during the first year	46 45	0.86
	Transfusion (n=205) No transfusion (n=218)	Patients with ≥ 1 rejection episodes during the first year	16 25	0.03
Sharma RK et al, 1997 §	DST (n=15) Non-DST (n=15)	Patient with biopsy-confirmed rejection episodes	4† 16†	< 0.01
	DST (n=15) Non-DST (n=15)	Patient with biopsy-confirmed rejection episodes	1.1‡ 0.26‡	< 0.01

*A transfusion was considered HLA-DR matched if a minimum of one HLA-DRB1 allele was present in the transfusion donor as well as recipient
† denotes total number of rejection episodes not percentage of patient with rejection episode
‡ denotes rejection rate per patient not percentage of patients with rejection episodes
§Rejection outcomes included in the above table provided some of the rejection endpoints that were evaluated in the study

DR=HLA-DR, DST=donor-specific transfusion, n=number of patients in the study group, NR=not reported, NS=not significant

Table 6. Results of good quality studies on graft survival

Study, Year	Intervention	Graft Survival Definition	1-year graft survival (%)	P-value	Max Duration	Max duration graftsurvival (%)	P-value
Marti HP et al, 2006	DST (n=55)	NR	98	NR	6 years	98	NR
	Control (n=55)		89			82	
Hiesse C et al, 2001a*	DR-matched transfusion (n=31)	NR	90	NR	5 years	79	NR
	No Transfusion (n=36)		92			80	
Hiesse C et al, 2001b*	DR-mismatched transfusion (n=39)	NR	92	NR	5 years	84	NR
	No Transfusion (n=36)		92			80	
Alexander JW, 1999	DST (n=115)	Death-censored graft survival	95	NR	2 years	90	NR
	Control (n=97)		95			90	
Opelz G et al, 1997*	Transfusion (n=205)	NR	90	0.02	5 years	79	0.03
	No Transfusion (n=218)		82			70	
Sharma RK et al, 1997	DST (n=15)	NR	86	> 0.05	1 year	86	> 0.05
	Non-DST (n=15)		75			75	

*Results of multivariate analyses were listed in Table 12

DR=HLA-DR, DST=donor-specific transfusion, n=number of patients in the study group, NR=not reported, NS=not significant

Table 7. Results of good quality studies on patient survival

Study, Year	Intervention	Patient Survival Definition	1-year patient survival (%)	P-value	Max Duration	Max duration patient survival (%)	P-value
Marti et al, 2006	DST (n=55)	NR	100	NR	6 years	100	NR
	Control (n=55)		100			93	
Hiesse C et al, 2001a	DR-matched transfusion (n=31)	NR	100	NS	5 years	86	NR
	No Transfusion (n=36)		100			92	
Hiesse C et al, 2001b	DR-mismatched transfusion (n=39)	NR	97	NS	5 years	97	NR
	No Transfusion (n=36)		100			92	
Alexander JW, 1999	DST (n=115)	NR	98	NR	2 years	97	NR
	Control (n=97)		100			98	
Opelz G et al, 1997	Transfusion (n=205)	NR	98	0.37	5 years	91	0.54
	No transfusion (n=218)		96			90	
Sharma RK et al, 1997	DST (n=15)	NR	92	NR	1 year	92	NR
	Non-DST (n=15)		86			86	

DR=HLA-DR, DST=donor-specific transfusion, n=number of patients in the study group, NR=not reported, NS=not significant

Figure 1. PRISMA Diagram

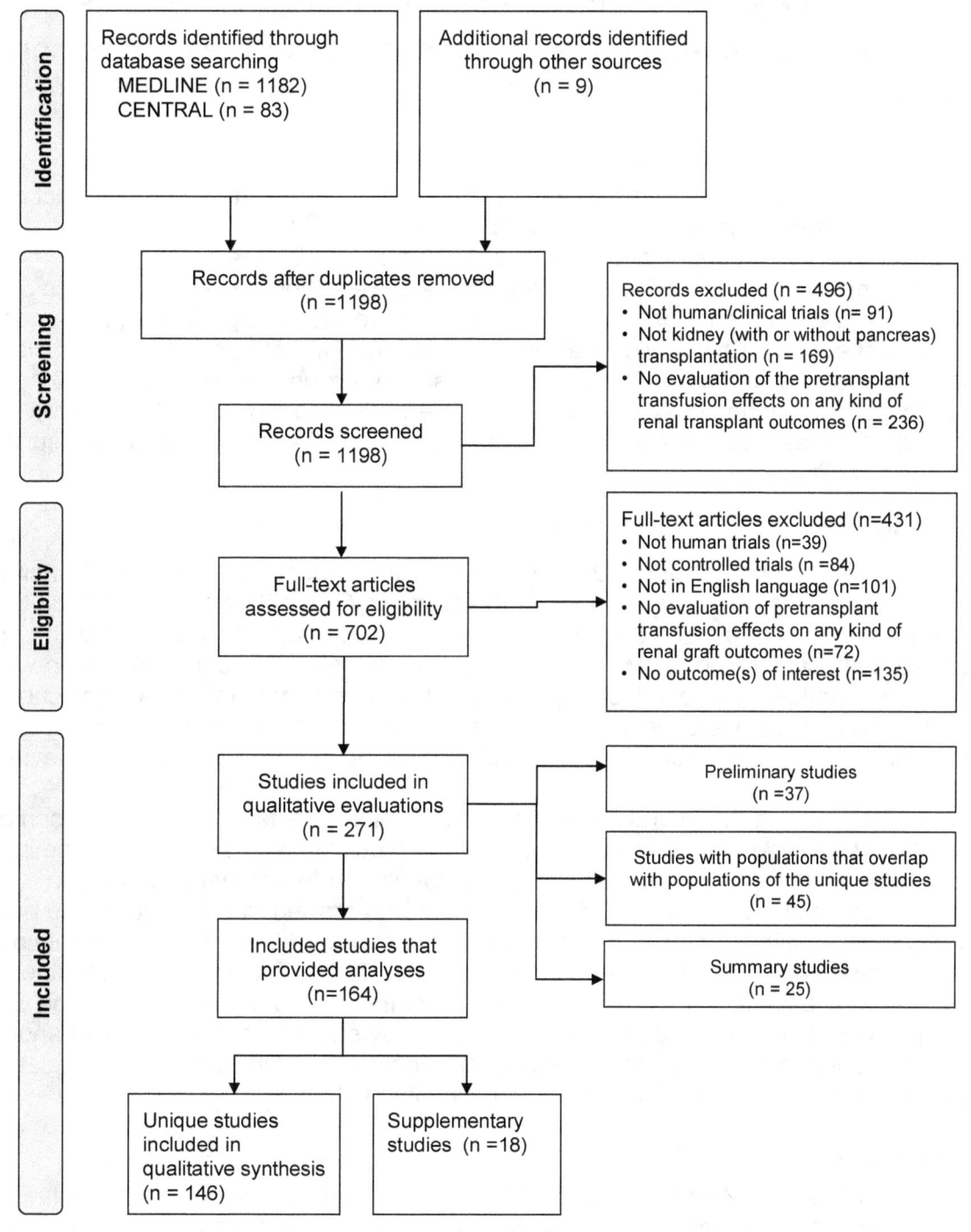

Key Question 1a. Do red blood cell transfusions prior to renal transplant impact allograft rejection/survival and what is the magnitude of that effect relative to other factors (e.g., pregnancy, prior transplantation?)

Univariate Analysis Results

One-hundred six unique studies were included in the evaluation of the impact of pretransplant transfusion on renal allograft outcomes.[14-81,81-119]

Nine of the 106 studies were clinical controlled trials, 12 were prospective observational studies, and 85 were retrospective observational studies, of which 5 (4.8 percent), 10 (9.4 percent), and 91 (85.8 percent) were rated as good, fair, and poor quality, respectively. Of the 401 analyses reported from the studies, 74 percent were from retrospective studies, with the remaining split between controlled trials (13 percent) and prospective studies (13 percent). Forty-seven (12 percent), 278 (69 percent), 76 (19 percent) analyses included results for graft rejection, graft survival and patient survival, respectively (Table 8).

Rejection [14-21,23,30,35,37,38,42,44,47,50,65,68-71,73,76,89,92,94,95,97,98,102-104,108,113,118]

Forty-seven analyses reported results on rejection outcomes, of which 25 analyses reported on the statistical significance of their results. Of the 25 analyses, 22 (88.0 percent) found either a significant reduction in rejection resulting from transfusion or no significant effect. To be considered in this evaluation, studies had to provide a p-value, 95 percent confidence interval, or explicitly say whether or not statistical significance was achieved. Thus, we concluded that transfusions had a significant beneficial to no significant effect on rejection outcomes and graded the strength of the body of evidence as low.

When evaluating the overall direction of transfusion effects on rejection outcomes, 36 of the 47 analyses (76.6 percent) found either a decreased risk or no change in rejection resulting from transfusion. Thus, we concluded that transfusions had a beneficial to neutral effect on rejection outcomes and graded the strength of the body of evidence as insufficient because in addition to the standard limitations within this body of evidence, it was difficult to gauge the magnitude of the effect from the available data (Table 9). To be classified as either decreasing or increasing the risk of rejection with transfusion, data had to be available within the study showing a direction of change or the text needed to note that the risk was either decreased or increased. Statistical significance was not evaluated in this directionality evaluation.

Graft Survival [14-20,22-45,47-68,70,72-86,88,90-120]

Fifty-five and sixty-five analyses performed statistical evaluations to determine if transfusions had a significant effect on 1-year and maximum duration graft survival, respectively. All available analyses reported either a significant increase or no significant effect on 1-year and maximum duration graft survival. None of the analyses found transfusion to have a significant negative impact on 1-year and maximum duration of graft survival. Thus, we concluded that transfusion had a significant beneficial to no significant effect on 1-year and maximum duration graft survival, and we graded the strength of the body of evidence for such effects to be low.

One-hundred thirty-two and one-hundred forty-six analyses performed evaluations of the magnitude of 1-year and maximum duration graft survival, respectively. One-hundred twenty-eight (96.9 percent) and one-hundred thirty-eight (94.5 percent) analyses reported either a >10 percent increase or a small change within 10 percent in either direction in survival on 1-year and maximum duration graft survival. Thus, we concluded that transfusion had a beneficial to neutral effect on 1-year and maximum duration graft survival, and we graded the strength of the body of evidence for such effects to be low (Table 10).

Patient Survival[14-18,23,29,33,37,38,50,53,59,62,65,71,77,86,88,89,93,95,99,104,106,108,111-113,118,120,121]

Sixteen and eighteen analyses performed statistical evaluations to determine if transfusions had a significant effect on 1-year and maximum duration patient survival, respectively. All available analyses reported either a significant increase or no significant effect on 1-year and maximum duration patient survival. None of the analyses found transfusion to have a significant negative impact on 1-year and maximum duration of patient survival. Thus, we concluded that transfusion has a significant beneficial to neutral effect on 1-year and maximum duration patient survival, and we graded the strength of the body of evidence for such effects to be low.

Thirty-five and forty-one analyses performed evaluations of the magnitude of 1-year and maximum duration patient survival, respectively. Thirty-three (94.3 percent) and thirty-seven (90.2 percent) analyses reported either a >10 percent increase or a small change within 10 percent in either direction in survival on 1-year and maximum duration patient survival. Thus, we concluded that transfusion has a beneficial to neutral effect on 1-year and maximum duration patient survival, and we graded the strength of the body of evidence for such effects to be low (Table 10).

Multivariate Analysis Results

Three analyses[122,123] evaluated prior transplantation as a covariate in multivariate analysis assessing for rejection. In two (66.7 percent) analyses, prior transplantations were independent predictors of increasing chances of rejection. The final analysis found that prior transplantation was not an independent predictor of rejection in either direction. Two analyses[113,123] evaluated prior transfusion as a covariate in multivariate analysis assessing for rejection. In both (100.0 percent) analyses, transfusions were independent predictors of decreasing rejection. One (100 percent) analysis[122] evaluated prior pregnancy as a covariate in multivariate analysis assessing for rejection. Prior pregnancy was an independent predictor of decreasing rejection (Table 11).

Twelve analyses[84,87,123-128] evaluated prior transplantation as a covariate in multivariate analysis assessing for graft survival. In six (50.0 percent) analyses, prior transplantations were independent predictor of worsening graft survival. The other analyses found that prior transplantations were not independent predictors of graft survival in either direction. Ten analyses[15,17,71,87,117,123,125,127] evaluated prior transfusion as a covariate in multivariate analysis assessing for graft survival. In five (50.0 percent) analyses,[124,126] transfusions were independent predictors of benefiting graft survival. The other analyses found that prior transfusions were not independent predictors of graft survival in either direction. Four analyses evaluated prior pregnancy as a covariate in multivariate analysis assessing for graft survival. In one (25.0 percent) analyses, pregnancy was an independent predictor of worsening graft survival. In this analysis, the covariate that was an independent predictor was three or more pregnancies. The other analyses found that prior pregnancies were not independent predictors of graft survival in either direction (Table 12).

Seven analyses[123,124,127,128] evaluated prior transplantation as a covariate in multivariate analysis assessing for patient survival. In one (14.3 percent) analysis, prior transplantation was an independent predictor of worsening patient survival. The other analyses found that prior transplantations were not independent predictors of patient survival in either direction. One analysis[127] evaluated prior transfusion as a covariate in multivariate analysis assessing for patient survival. This analysis found that prior transplantation was not an independent predictor of patient survival in either direction. No analyses evaluated prior pregnancy as a covariate in multivariate analysis assessing for patient survival (Table 13).

In summary, prior transplant may induce increases in rejection and worsening graft survival or no significant changes may occur in these outcomes but benefits are unlikely to result from these outcomes. Transfusions may be related to decreasing rejection and benefiting graft survival or no significant changes may occur but it is unlikely that these outcomes would worsen as a result of transfusion. Prior pregnancy had very scant data and could not be well assessed.

Table 8. Insight into body of literature: Transfusion versus no transfusion (KQ 1a)

	Rejection	Graft Survival	Patient Survival	Validity of Studies
KQ 1a. Transfusion versus No transfusion	CCT 9 Analyses	CCT 1-year – 12 Analyses Max time – 13 Analyses	CCT 1-year – 8 Analyses Max time – 8 Analyses	Good 5 studies
	POBS 1 Analysis	POBS 1-year – 24 Analyses Max time – 27 Analyses	POBS 1-year – 1 Analysis Max time – 3 Analyses	Fair 10 studies
	ROBS 37 Analyses	ROBS 1-year – 96 Analyses Max time – 106 Analyses	ROBS 1-year – 26 Analyses Max time – 30 Analyses	Poor 91 studies

CCT=clinical controlled trial, KQ=key question, Max=maximum followup time, POBS=prospective observational studies, ROBS=retrospective observational studies

Table 9. Impact of transfusions (any type) on rejection (KQ 1a)

Impact of Transfusions on:	Significant Reduction in Rejection	No Significant Effect on Rejection	Significant Increases in Rejection	Decreased Risk of Rejection*	No Change in Rejection†	Increased Risk of Rejection*

Impact of Transfusions on:	Significant Reduction in Rejection	No Significant Effect on Rejection	Significant Increases in Rejection	Decreased Risk of Rejection*	No Change in Rejection†	Increased Risk of Rejection*
Rejection at Any Time Point	9/25 (36.0%)	13/25 (52.0%)	3/25 (12.0%)	28/47 (59.6%)	8/47 (17.0%)	11/47 (23.4%)

*Data either showing a decrease/increase of any magnitude or notation in text stating a decrease/increase
†Data either showing no difference, or notation in text stating no change

Table 10. Impact of transfusions (any type) on graft and patient survival (KQ1a)

Impact of transfusions on:	Significant Increases in Survival	No Significant Effect	Significant Decreases in Survival	>10% Increase in Survival	10% to -10% Change in Survival	>10% Decrease in Survival
1-Year Graft Survival	29/55 (52.7%)	26/55 (47.3%)	0/55 (0.0%)	65/132 (49.2%)	63/132 (47.7%)	4/132 (3.1%)
Max Duration Graft Survival	30/65 (46.2%)	35/65 (53.8%)	0/65 (0.0%)	76/146 (52.0%)	62/146 (42.5%)	8/146 (5.5%)
1-Year Patient Survival	0/16 (0.0%)	16/16 (100%)	0/16 (0.0%)	1/35 (2.9%)	32/35 (91.4%)	2/35 (5.7%)
Max Duration Patient Survival	1/18 (5.6%)	17/18 (94.4%)	0/18 (0.0%)	8/41 (19.5%)	29/41 (70.7%)	4/41 (9.8%)

Table 11. Multivariate results: the impact of transfusions on rejection (KQ 1a)

Study, Year Total N	Analysis Type	Covariate	Outcome Evaluated	Multivariate Results	Significant Effect
Impact of previous transplant					
Reed A, 1991 N=127	Poisson*	Prior transplant	Rejection episodes	NR, P=0.40	NA
Sanfilippo F, 1986 N=3811	Cox†	Prior failed graft (1)	Irreversible graft rejection	RR 1.409, P=0.0002	Transplant worsens rejection
Sanfilippo F, 1986 N=3811	Cox†	Prior failed grafts (≥2)	Irreversible graft rejection	RR 1.884, P=0.0006	Transplant worsens rejection
Impact of pretransplant transfusions					
Waanders MM, 2008 N=118	Cox†	Pretransplant protocol blood transfusion	Severe acute rejection	HR 0.385 (0.186-0.796), P=0.010	Transfusion benefits rejection
Sanfilippo F, 1986 N=3811	Cox†	No pretransplant transfusion	Irreversible graft rejection	RR 1.377, P=0.0003	Transfusion benefits rejection
Impact of pregnancy					
Reed A, 1991 N=127	Poisson*	Pregnancy	Rejection episodes	NR, P=0.017	Pregnancy benefits rejection

* Poisson multivariate analysis
† Cox proportional hazards regression analysis
HR=hazard ratio; N=number of patients in analysis; NR=not reported; NS=not significant; RR=relative risk

Table 12. Multivariate results: the impact of transfusions on graft survival (KQ1a)

Study, Year Total N	Analysis Type	Covariate	Outcome Evaluated	Multivariate Results	Significant Effect
Impact of previous transplant					
Tang H, 2008 N=2882	Cox*	Previous transplant	Graft failure	HR 2.29 (1.73-3.02), P<0.001	Transplant worsens graft survival
Peters TG, 1995 Study period: 1982-1991 N=17,937	Cox*	Retransplant	Graft survival	RR 1.35, P<0.0001	Transplant worsens graft survival
Poli F, 1995 N=416	Cox*	Graft number (first transplant, re-transplant)	Graft survival	RR 1.4 (0.5-4.0), P=0.3	NA
Sautner T, 1994 N=146	Stepwise logistic regression	History of prior transplants (1)	Graft loss	RR 1.4, P=0.005	Transplant worsens graft survival
Sautner T, 1994 N=146	Stepwise logistic regression	History of prior transplants (≥2)	Graft loss	RR 0.21x10^5, P=0.005	Transplant worsens graft survival
Madrenas J, 1988 N=287	Cox*	Second transplant	Graft survival	RR 1.179, P=NS	NA
Madrenas J, 1988 N=287	Cox*	≥3 transplants	Graft survival	RR 1.606, P=NS	NA
CMTSG, 1986 CyA[†] N=142	Cox*	Prior transplant	Graft loss	RR 0.60, P=NS	NA
CMTSG, 1986 Control[‡] N=149	Cox*	Prior transplant	Graft loss	RR 1.33, P=NS	NA
Sanfilippo F, 1986 N=3811	Cox*	Prior failed graft (1)	Graft failure	RR 1.217, P=0.011	Transplant worsens graft survival
Sanfilippo F, 1986 N=3811	Cox*	Prior failed grafts (≥2)	Graft failure	RR 1.506, P=0.009	Transplant worsens graft survival
Rao KV, 1983 N=300	Cox*	Previous transplants	Graft survival	NR, P=0.3380	NA
Impact of pretransplant transfusions					

Study, Year Total N	Analysis Type	Covariate	Outcome Evaluated	Multivariate Results	Significant Effect
Lietz K, 2003 N=502	Cox*	Blood transfusions	Graft survival	RR 1.316 (0.671-2.582), P=0.4243	NA
Hiesse C, 2001 N=144	Cox*	No transfusion (vs. matched or mis-matched transfusion)	Graft survival	HR 1.1 (0.51-2.48), P=0.76	NA
Hiesse C, 2001 N=144	Cox*	Transfusion with 1-DR matched blood	Graft survival	HR 0.59 (0.22-1.55), P=0.28	NA
Opelz G, 1997 N=423	Cox*	Pretransplant transfusions – 1 year f/u	Graft survival	RR 2.5, P=0.003	Transfusion benefits graft survival
Opelz G, 1997 N=423	Cox*	Pretransplant transfusions – 5 year f/u	Graft survival	RR 1.9, P=0.006	Transfusion benefits graft survival
Peters TG, 1995 Study period: 1982-1991 N=17,937	Cox*	Pre-transplant transfusions	Graft survival	RR 0.79, P<0.0001	Transfusion benefits graft survival
Xiao X, 1992 N=201	Cox*	Pretransplant transfusion	Graft survival	RR 0.9998, P=0.128	NA
Madrenas J, 1988 N=287	Cox*	Pretransplant blood transfusions	Graft survival	RR 0.5447, P=0.018	Transfusion benefits graft survival
Sanfilippo F, 1986 N=3811	Cox*	No pretransplant transfusion	Graft failure	RR 1.321, P=0.0002	Transfusion benefits graft survival
Rao KV, 1983 N=300	Cox*	Blood transfusions	Graft survival	NR, P=0.2765	NA
Impact of pregnancy					
Tang H, 2008 Females only N=2349	Cox*	Pregnancy (1)	Graft failure	HR 1.11 (0.79-1.56), P=0.554	NA
Tang H, 2008 Females only N=2349	Cox*	Pregnancies (2)	Graft failure	HR 1.28 (0.91-1.81), P=0.147	NA

Study, Year Total N	Analysis Type	Covariate	Outcome Evaluated	Multivariate Results	Significant Effect
Tang H, 2008 Females only N=2349	Cox*	Pregnancies (≥3)	Graft failure	HR 1.54 (1.11-2.16), P<0.05	Pregnancy worsens graft survival
Sautner T, 1994 N=146	Stepwise logistic regression	Pregnancies	Graft survival	NR, P=NS	NA

* Cox proportional hazards regression analysis
† Patients received immunosuppression with cyclosporine
‡ Patients received control immunosuppression with azathioprine
CyA=cyclosporine; CMTSG=Canadian Multicenter Transplant Study Group; f/u=followup; HR=hazard ratio; N=number of patients in analysis; NR=not reported; NS=not significant; RR=relative risk

Table 13. Multivariate results: the impact of transfusions on patient survival (KQ1a)

Study, Year Total N	Analysis Type	Covariate	Outcome Evaluated	Multivariate Results	Significant Effect
Impact of previous transplant					
Tang H, 2008 N=2882	Cox*	Previous transplant	Patient death	HR 3.59 (2.69-4.80), P<0.001	Transplant worsens patient survival
Madrenas J, 1988 N=287	Cox*	Second transplant	Patient survival	RR 1.261, P=NS	NA
Madrenas J, 1988 N=287	Cox*	≥3 transplants	Patient survival	RR 3.968, P=NS	NA
CMTSG, 1986 CyA N=142	Cox*	Prior transplant	Patient death	RR 0.49, P=NS	NA
CMTSG, 1986 Control N=149	Cox*	Prior transplant	Patient death	RR 1.10, P=NS	NA
Sanfilippo F, 1986 N=3811	Cox*	Prior failed graft (1)	Patient death	RR 0.998, P=NS	NA
Sanfilippo F, 1986 N=3811	Cox*	Prior failed grafts (≥2)	Patient death	RR 1.712, P=0.08	NA

Study, Year Total N	Analysis Type	Covariate	Outcome Evaluated	Multivariate Results	Significant Effect
Impact of pretransplant transfusions					
Madrenas J, 1988 N=287	Cox*	Pretransplant blood transfusions	Patient survival	RR 0.7447, P=NS	NA

* Cox proportional hazards regression analysis
CMTSG=Canadian Multicenter Transplant Study Group; HR=hazard ratio; N=number of patients in analysis; NA=not applicable; NR=not reported; NS=not significant; RR=relative risk

Evaluation of Different Types of Transfusions on Renal Allograft Outcomes

While our base-case analyses combined different types of transfusions to assess the overall impact of transfusion on renal transplant outcomes, in these subgroup evaluations, we separated the analyses of donor-specific transfusions versus no transfusion from other types of transfusions versus no transfusion.

Non-DST Therapeutic/Protocol Transfusions [15,17,19,20,24-29,31-37,39-45,48,49,51-58,60-63,65,66,69,71-76,78-88,90,91,95,96,98,100-103,105-107,109-111,113-117,119,120,129]

Of the 106 unique studies included in Key Question 1a, 267 analyses reported the impact of therapeutic or protocol transfusion on renal allograft outcomes. Of the 267 analyses, 20 (7.5 percent),[15,17,19,20,35,37,42,44,65,69,71,73,76,95,98,102,103,113] 204 (76.4 percent),[15,17,19,20,24-29,31-37,39-45,48,49,51-58,60-63,65,66,72-86,88,90,91,95,96,98,100-103,105-107,109-111,113-117,119,120,130] and 43 (16.1 percent) analyses[15,17,29,33,37,53,62,65,71,77,86,88,95,103,106,111,113,120] included results for rejection, graft survival and patient survival respectively (Table 14).

Fourteen of the twenty analyses provided statistical significance of the results on graft rejection, of which 12 (86 percent) found therapeutic or protocol transfusions to have significant beneficial to no significant effect on rejection outcomes. The strength of body of evidence of this outcome was graded as low. For the overall direction of therapeutic or protocol transfusion effects on rejection outcomes, eighty-five percent of the analyses found such transfusions to have beneficial to neutral effect, and we graded the strength of evidence as insufficient because the magnitude of the effect from the available data was difficult to gauge (Table 15).

All the analyses that reported significance of results on both graft and patient survival found that therapeutic or protocol transfusions either significantly improved or had no significant effect on survival outcomes at 1-year and maximum duration. The vast majority (83 to 96 percent) of analyses found the magnitude of the transfusion effects on graft and patient survival at 1-year and maximum duration to be beneficial or neutral (Table 16). The strength of the body of evidence in all cases was low.

The results of this subgroup analysis were not markedly different from those of our base-case analyses, thus the overall conclusion for Key Question 1a remains the same.

Table 14. Insight into body of literature: *therapeutic/protocol transfusions versus no transfusion (excluding DST analyses)* (KQ 1a)

	Rejection	Graft Survival	Patient survival	Validity of Studies
KQ 1a. Transfusion versus No transfusion	CCT 4 Analyses	CCT 1-year –8 Analyses Max time –8 Analyses	CCT 1-year –3 Analyses Max time –3 Analyses	Good 2 studies
	POBS 0 Analysis	POBS 1-year –16 Analyses Max time –19 Analyses	POBS 1-year –0 Analysis Max time –2 Analyses	Fair 5 studies

	Rejection	Graft Survival	Patient survival	Validity of Studies
	ROBS	ROBS	ROBS	Poor
	16 Analyses	1-year –75 Analyses	1-year –17 Analyses	73 studies
		Max time –78 Analyses	Max time –18 Analyses	

Abbreviations: CCT=clinical controlled trial, KQ=key question, Max=maximum followup time, POBS=prospective observational studies, ROBS=retrospective observational studies

Table 15. Impact of *therapeutic/protocol transfusions (excluding DST analyses)* on rejection (KQ 1a)

Impact of transfusions on:	Significant Reduction in Rejection	No Significant Effect on Rejection	Significant Increases in Rejection	Decreased Risk of Rejection*	No Change in Rejection †	Increased Risk of Rejection*
Rejection at Any Time Point	6/14 (42.9%)	6/14 (42.9%)	2/14 (14.2%)	13/20 (65.0%)	4/20 (20.0%)	3/20 (15.0%)

*Data either showing a decrease/increase of any magnitude or notation in text stating a decrease/increase
†Data either showing no difference, or notation in text stating no change

Table 16. Impact of *therapeutic/protocol transfusion (excluding DST analyses)* on graft and patient survival (KQ1a)

Impact of transfusions on:	Significant Increases in Survival	No Significant Effect	Significant Decreases in Survival	>10% Increase in Survival	10% to -10% Change in Survival	>10% Decrease in Survival
1-Year Graft Survival	22/43 (51.2%)	21/43 (48.8%)	0/43 (0.0%)	54/99 (54.5%)	41/99 (41.4%)	4/99 (4.1%)
Max Duration Graft Survival	21/47 (44.7%)	26/47 (55.3%)	0/47 (0.0%)	58/105 (55.2%)	41/105 (39.0%)	6/105 (5.7%)
1-Year Patient Survival	0/12 (0.0%)	12/12 (100%)	0/12 (0.0%)	1/20 (5.0%)	17/20 (85.0%)	2/20 (10.0%)
Max Duration Patient Survival	1/12 (8.3%)	11/12 (91.7%)	0/12 (0.0%)	4/23 (17.4%)	15/23 (65.2%)	4/23 (17.4%)

Donor-Specific Transfusion[14,16,18,19,21-23,30,32,38,47,50,51,59,64,65,67,68,70,89,92-97,99,104,108,112,118]

Thirty-one of the 106 unique studies included in Key Question 1a evaluated the impact of donor specific transfusions on renal allograft outcomes. A total of 134 analyses were reported in the DST studies, of which 27, 74, and 33 analyses were included for rejection outcomes, graft and patient survival, respectively. (Table 17)

A little over 90 percent of the analyses that reported the significance of results on rejection outcomes found that DST either significantly reduced or had no significant effect on rejection. Although DST was shown to have more beneficial effects (56 percent) on rejection outcomes when assessing the direction of its effect, 30 percent of the total rejection analyses also found DST to have detrimental effects on graft rejection. As such, 70 percent of the analyses found either a beneficial or neutral effect on graft rejection. The strength of the body of evidence for the significance of results on rejection was low, while the strength of evidence for the magnitude of DST effects was graded as insufficient. (Table 18)

All analyses that reported significance results of graft survival found that DST either significantly improved or had no significant effect on 1-year and maximum duration of graft survival, while all analyses found DST to have no significant effect on 1-year and maximum duration of patient survival. For the magnitude of DST effects, the use of DST was found to have a beneficial or neutral effect on graft and patient survival in 95–100% of analyses at 1-year and maximum duration of followup. The strength of evidence in all cases was low. (Table 19)

Table 17. Insight into body of literature: *DST versus no transfusion* (KQ 1a)

	Rejection	Graft Survival	Patient survival	Validity of Studies
KQ 1a. Transfusion versus No transfusion	CCT 5 Analyses	CCT 1-year –4 Analyses Max time –5 Analyses	CCT 1-year –5 Analyses Max time –5 Analyses	Good 3 studies
	POBS 1 Analysis	POBS 1-year –8 Analyses Max time –8 Analyses	POBS 1-year –1 Analysis Max time –1 Analyses	Fair 8 studies
	ROBS 21 Analyses	ROBS 1-year –21 Analyses Max time –28 Analyses	ROBS 1-year –9 Analyses Max time –12 Analyses	Poor 19 studies

Abbreviations: CCT=clinical controlled trial, KQ=key question, Max=maximum followup time, POBS=prospective observational studies, ROBS=retrospective observational studies

Table 18. Impact of *DST* on rejection (KQ 1a)

Impact of transfusions on:	Significant Reduction in Rejection	No Significant Effect on Rejection	Significant Increases in Rejection	Decreased Risk of Rejection*	No Change in Rejection[†]	Increased Risk of Rejection*
Rejection at Any Time Point	3/11	7/11	1/11	15/27	4/27	8/27

| | (27.3%) | (63.6%) | (9.1%) | (55.6%) | (14.8%) | (29.6%) |

*Data either showing a decrease/increase of any magnitude or notation in text stating a decrease/increase
†Data either showing no difference, or notation in text stating no change

Table 19. Impact of *DST* on graft and patient survival (KQ1a)

Impact of transfusions on:	Significant Increases in Survival	No Significant Effect	Significant Decreases in Survival	>10% Increase in Survival	10% to -10% Change in Survival	>10% Decrease in Survival
1-Year Graft Survival	7/12 (58.3%)	5/12 (41.7%)	0/12 (0.0%)	11/33 (33.3%)	22/33 (66.7%)	0/33 (0.0%)
Max Duration Graft Survival	9/18 (50.0%)	9/18 (50.0%)	0/18 (0.0%)	18/41 (43.9%)	21/41 (51.2%)	2/41 (4.9%)
1-Year Patient Survival	0/4 (0.0%)	4/4 (100%)	0/4 (0.0%)	0/15 (0.0%)	15/15 (100.0%)	0/15 (0.0%)
Max Duration Patient Survival	0/6 (0.0%)	6/6 (100.0%)	0/6 (0.0%)	4/18 (22.2%)	14/18 (77.8%)	0/18 (0.0%)

Key Question 1bi. Is any such impact of red blood cell transfusions on renal transplant outcomes altered by planned DST versus therapeutic transfusions?

Univariate Analysis Results

Eleven unique studies were included in the evaluation of the impact of planned DST versus non-DST on renal transplant outcomes.[32,51,65,96,122,131-136] One of the 11 studies was a prospective observational study, and 10 were retrospective observational studies, of which 2 (18.2 percent) were rated as fair quality and 9 (81.8 percent) were rated as poor quality. Of the 48 analyses reported from the studies, 25 percent were from the prospective study, and 75 percent were from retrospective studies. Seven (14.5 percent), 33 (68.8 percent), and 8 (16.7 percent) included results for graft rejection, graft survival and patient survival, respectively (Table 20).

Rejection[65,122,131-133,136]

Seven analyses reported results on rejection outcomes of which three (42.8 percent) analyses reported on the statistical significance of the results. These three analyses found either a significant reduction in rejection or no significant effect associated with DST.[65,122,136] To be considered in this evaluation, studies had to provide a p-value, 95 percent confidence interval, or explicitly state whether or not statistical significance was achieved. Thus, we concluded that planned DST had a significant beneficial to neutral effect on rejection outcomes and graded the strength of the body of evidence as low. When assessing the overall direction of change for DST versus non-DST on rejection outcomes, six of seven analyses (85.8 percent) found either a decreased risk or no change in rejection resulting from planned DST. We concluded that DST versus non-DST had a beneficial to neutral impact on rejection outcomes. We graded the strength of evidence as insufficient as it was challenging to gauge the magnitude of the effect from the available data. (Table 21) To be classified as either decreasing or increasing the risk of rejection with transfusion, data had to be available within the study showing a direction of change or the text needed to note that the risk was either decreased or increased. Statistical significance was not evaluated in this directionality evaluation.

Graft Survival[65,131,132,135,136]

Four and five analyses completed statistical evaluations to determine if DST had a significant effect on 1-year and maximum duration graft survival, respectively (Table 22). All presented analyses determined that DST had either a significant increase or no significant effect on 1-year and maximum duration graft survival. None of the analyses found DST to have a negative significant impact on 1-year and maximum duration graft survival. Therefore, we concluded that DST versus non-DST had a beneficial to neutral significant effect on 1-year and maximum duration graft survival. The strength of evidence was graded as low.

Sixteen and seventeen analyses evaluated the magnitude of 1-year and maximum duration graft survival, respectively. All analyses reported either a >10 percent increase or a small change within 10 percent in either direction in survival with regard to 1-year and maximum duration graft survival. We concluded that DST had a beneficial to neutral effect on 1-year and maximum duration graft survival, and that the strength of evidence for these effects to be low.

Patient Survival[65,133,135]

Two analyses and two analyses performed statistical evaluations to establish if DST had a significant effect on 1-year and maximum duration patient survival, respectively (Table 22). All analyses demonstrated that DST had no significant effect on 1-year and maximum duration patient survival. None of the analysis found DST to have a significant increase or decrease in 1-year and maximum patient survival. We concluded that DST versus non-DST had no significant effect on 1-year and maximum duration patient survival. We graded the strength of evidence for these effects to be insufficient.

Four analyses and four analyses examined the extent of DST on 1-year and maximum duration patient survival, respectively. All analyses reported a small change within 10 percent in either direction on 1-year and maximum duration patient survival. We concluded that DST versus non-DST had a neutral effect on 1-year and maximum duration patient survival, and we assessed the strength of the body of evidence for these effects to be low.

Multivariate Analysis Results

One analysis[122] evaluated DST as a covariate in multivariate analysis assessing for rejection episodes (Table 23). DST was found to be an independent predictor of decreasing rejection in this analysis.

Four analyses[64,96] evaluated the effects of DST for graft survival in multivariate analyses. One of the four analyses (25.0 percent) found that DST was an independent predictor in benefiting graft survival. The other analyses did not find that DST was an independent predictor. However, in three of the four analyses, including the one in which it was found to be an independent predictor, DST was compared to no transfusion, not to a non-DST transfusion. No analysis examined DST as a covariate in multivariate analysis evaluating patient survival (Table 24).

In summary, DST may or may not impact rejection, may or may not benefit graft survival and the impact on patient survival is unknown.

Table 20. Insight into body of literature: Donor-specific transfusion (KQ 1bi)

	Rejection	Graft Survival	Patient survival	Validity of Studies
KQ 1bi. DST	CCT None	CCT None	CCT None	Good None
	POBS None	POBS 1-year – 6 Analyses Max time – 6 Analyses	POBS None	Fair 2 studies
	ROBS 7 Analyses	ROBS 1-year – 10 Analyses Max time – 11 Analyses	ROBS 1-year – 4 Analyses Max time – 4 Analyses	Poor 9 studies

CCT=clinical controlled trial, DST=donor specific transfusion, KQ=key question, Max=maximum followup time, POBS=prospective observational studies, ROBS=retrospective observational studies

Table 21. Impact of donor specific transfusion on rejection (KQ1bi)

KQ 1bi	Significant Decreases in Rejection	No Significant Effect on Rejection	Significant Increases in Rejection	Decreased Risk of Rejection*	No Change in Rejection†	Increased Risk of Rejection*
Graft Rejection Any Time Point	2/3 (66.7%)	1/3 (33.3%)	0/3 (0.0%)	3/7 (42.9%)	3/7 (42.9%)	1/7 (14.2%)

*Data either showing a decrease/increase o00f any magnitude or notation in text stating a decrease/increase
†Data either showing no difference, or notation in text stating no change

Table 22. Impact of DST on graft and patient survival (KQ 1bi)

KQ 1bi	Significant Increases in Survival	No Significant Effect	Significant Decreases in Survival	>10% Increase in Survival	10% to -10% Change in Survival	>10% Decrease in Survival
1-Year Graft Survival	2/4 (50.0%)	2/4 (50.0%)	0/4 (0.0%)	3/16 (18.8%)	13/16 (81.2%)	0/16 (0.0%)
Max Duration Graft Survival	2/5 (40.0%)	3/5 (60.0%)	0/5 (0.0%)	6/17 (35.3%)	11/17 (64.7%)	0/17 (0.0%)
1-Year Patient Survival	0/2 (0%)	2/2 (100%)	0/2 (0%)	0/4 (0%)	4/4 (100%)	0/4 (0%)

KQ 1bi	Significant Increases in Survival	No Significant Effect	Significant Decreases in Survival	>10% Increase in Survival	10% to -10% Change in Survival	>10% Decrease in Survival
Max Duration Patient Survival	0/2 (0%)	2/2 (100%)	0/2 (0%)	0/4 (0%)	4/4 (100%)	0/4 (0%)

Table 23. Multivariate results: Impact of DST on rejection (KQ1bi)

Study, Year Total N	Analysis Type	Covariate	Outcome Evaluated	Multivariate Results	Significant Effect
Reed A, 1991 N=127	Poisson multivariate analysis	DST	Rejection episodes	NR, P=0.0001	DST benefits rejection

DST=donor specific transfusion; N=number of patients in analysis; NR=not reported

Table 24. Multivariate results: Impact of DST on graft survival (KQ bi)

Study, Year Total N	Analysis Type	Covariate	Outcome Evaluated	Multivariate Results	Significant Effect
Jin DC, 1996 N=680	Cox*	DST	Graft survival	RR 0.808, P=0.2729	NA
Sanfilippo F, 1990 N=2138	Cox*	DST vs. no transfusion	Graft survival	RR 0.77, P=NS	NA
Sanfilippo F, 1990 1-haplotype match N=1246	Cox*	DST vs. no transfusion	Graft survival	RR 0.56, P<0.06	DST benefits graft survival
Sanfilippo F, 1990 2-haplotype match N=750	Cox*	DST vs. no transfusion	Graft survival	RR 1.03, P=NS	NA

* Cox proportional hazards regression analysis
DST=donor specific transfusion; N=number of patients in analysis; NS=not significant; RR=relative risk

Key Question 1bii. Is any such impact of red blood cell transfusions on renal transplant outcomes altered by the number of transfusions, the number of units of blood, and/or the number of donors?

Univariate Analysis Results

We answered this key question by categorizing the number of transfusions and the number of units of blood into four groups: zero, 1 to ≤5, 5 to 10 (or ≥ 5), and ≥ 10 transfusions or units of blood. Pairwise comparisons of different transfusion intensities (i.e. transfusion intensities versus no transfusion and higher intensity versus lower intensity) were conducted to evaluate whether transfusion effects on survival outcomes would be altered by the number of transfusions or units of blood transfused.

Thirty-seven unique studies were included in the evaluation of the impact of different number of transfusions on renal allograft outcomes.[3,20,24,34,37,41,43,45,52,57,64,72,73,98,101,102,106,109,115,116,119,126,128,137-150] Three of the 37 studies were clinical controlled trials, two were prospective observational studies, and 32 were retrospective observational studies, of which none was rated as good quality, 7 rated fair, and 30 rated poor. Of the 314 analyses reported by the studies, the majority of analyses (88.4 percent) were from retrospective studies, while only 6.8 percent and 4.8 percent of the analyses were from controlled trials and prospective studies respectively. Nineteen (6.1 percent), 265 (84.3 percent), and 30 (9.6 percent) analyses included results for graft rejection, graft survival and patient survival, respectively (Table 25).

Rejection

Number of transfusions[37,73,102,138]

Eighteen analyses reported results on rejection outcomes, of which 5 of the 18 analyses reported on the statistical significance of their results. Of the five analyses, all found either a significant reduction in rejection resulting from using any higher versus any lower number of transfusions or no significant effect. To be considered in this evaluation, studies had to provide a p-value, 95 percent confidence interval, or explicitly say whether or not statistical significance was achieved. Thus, we concluded that the use of larger number of transfusions had a beneficial to no significant effect on rejection outcomes and graded the strength of the body of evidence as low (Table 26).

When evaluating the overall direction of transfusion effects on rejection outcomes, 16 of the 18 analyses (88.9 percent) found either a decreased risk or no change in rejection resulting from using any higher versus any lower number of transfusions. Thus, we concluded that any higher number of transfusions had a beneficial to neutral effect on rejection outcomes and graded the strength of the body of evidence as insufficient because in addition to the standard limitations within this body of evidence, it was difficult to gauge the magnitude of the effect from the available data (Table 26). To be classified as either decreasing or increasing the risk of rejection with transfusion, data had to be available within the study showing a direction of change or the text needed to note that the risk was either decreased or increased. Statistical significance was not evaluated in this directionality evaluation.

Units of Transfusions[20]

One analysis reported results on rejection outcomes of which it found no significant effect on rejection outcomes. The direction of transfusion effects resulting from using any higher number versus any lower number of units of blood did not change rejection outcomes. Thus, we concluded that the use of any number of units of blood had a neutral effect on rejection outcomes and graded the strength of the body of evidence as insufficient. In addition to the standard limitations within this body of evidence, it was difficult to gauge the magnitude of the effect from the available data (Table 26). To be classified as either decreasing or increasing the risk of rejection with transfusion, data had to be available within the study showing a direction of change or the text needed to note that the risk was either decreased or increased. Statistical significance was not evaluated in this directionality evaluation.

Number of donors

No analysis reported results on rejection outcomes. Thus, there was insufficient data to grade the strength of evidence on the effect of number of donors on graft rejection.

Graft Survival

Number of transfusions[3,34,37,41,57,73,98,101,102,106,109,115,116,126,128,137,138,140-146,150]

Any number of transfusions versus no transfusion

Twelve and nine analyses performed statistical evaluations to determine if different number of transfusions had a significant effect on 1- year and maximum duration graft survival versus no transfusions, respectively. The comparisons were made between different intensity of transfusions versus no transfusions (1-5, 5-10, and ≥10 transfusions versus no transfusions). Receiving 1 to 5 or ten or more transfusions had only significantly beneficial or no significant effects of 1-year and maximal duration graft survival versus no transfusions. While two analyses found that 5-10 transfusions had a significant beneficial effect on 1-year and maximal duration graft survival versus no transfusions, two analyses (one for 1-year and the other for maximum duration), both reported in the same study by Chavers et al, found receiving more than five transfusions to have significant detrimental effect on 1-year and maximum duration graft survival versus no transfusion.[138] Another analysis found >5 transfusion versus no transfusion to have a significant negative effect on maximum duration graft survival.[126] In a final analysis of 1-year graft survival, >5-10 transfusions versus no transfusion was found to have no significant effect on graft survival. Thus, we concluded that having 1-5 and ten or more transfusions has a beneficial to no significant effect on 1-year and maximum duration graft survival versus no transfusions, the impact of 5-10 transfusions is mixed, and we graded the strength of the body of evidence for such effects to be low (Table 27).

Fifty-one and fifty-three analyses performed evaluations of the magnitude of 1-year and maximum duration graft survival for different numbers of transfusions (1-5, 5-10, and ≥10 transfusions) versus no transfusions, respectively. Forty-nine (96.1 percent) and forty-nine (92.5 percent) analyses reported either a >10 percent increase or a small change within 10 percent in either direction in survival on 1-year and maximum duration graft survival, respectively. Thus, we concluded that different number of transfusion has a beneficial to neutral effect on 1-year and maximum duration graft survival, and we graded the strength of the body of evidence for such effects to be low.

Higher number versus lower number of transfusions

Eleven and ten analyses performed statistical evaluations to determine if higher versus lower number of blood transfusions had a significant effect on 1-year and maximum duration graft survival, respectively. For 1-year survival, nine of the eleven (82 percent) analyses in the three different pairwise groups (>5 versus 1-5, >10 versus 1-5, >10 versus 5-10) reported either a significant increase or no significant effect on 1-year graft survival. Two of the 11 analyses (18 percent) found > 5 transfusions versus 1-5 transfusions to have a significant negative impact on 1-year graft survival. For maximum duration, only the evaluation of >5 versus 1-5 transfusions had evaluable analyses, of which 7 out of 11 (64 percent) analyses found a significant beneficial or no significant effect. The remaining four analyses (36 percent) found >5 transfusions to have a significant negative impact on maximum duration of graft survival. Thus, we concluded that different number of transfusions has a beneficial to no significant effect on 1-year and maximum duration graft survival, and we graded the strength of the body of evidence for such effects to be low to insufficient (Table 28).

Forty-three and forty-seven analyses performed evaluations of the magnitude of 1-year and maximum duration graft survival for higher versus lower number of blood transfusions, respectively. For 1-year survival, all available analyses in the three different pairwise groups (>5 versus 1-5, >10 versus 1-5, >10 versus 5-10) reported either a >10 percent increase or a small change within 10 percent in either direction on 1-year and maximum duration graft survival. For maximum duration, in 42 of 47 analyses (89.4 percent), a beneficial or neutral effect was seen with higher versus lower number of transfusions. Thus, we concluded that different number of transfusion has a beneficial to neutral effect on 1-year and maximum duration graft survival, and we graded the strength of the body of evidence for such effects to be low.

Units of transfusions[20,24,43,45,52,64,72,119,139,148,149]

Any units of transfusions versus no transfusion

Eleven and sixteen analyses performed statistical evaluations to determine if different number of units transfused had a significant effect on 1- year and maximum duration graft survival versus no transfusions, respectively. The comparisons were made between different intensity of units transfused versus no units (1-5 versus 0, 5-10 versus 0, and ≥10 versus 0 transfusions). All available analyses in three different pairwise groups reported either a significant beneficial or no significant effect on 1-year and maximum duration graft survival. None of the analyses found the number of units transfused to have a significant negative impact on 1-year and maximum duration of graft survival. Thus, we concluded that different number of units transfused has a beneficial to no significant effect on 1-year and maximum duration graft survival, and we graded the strength of the body of evidence for such effects to be low (Table 29).

Twenty-one and twenty-two analyses performed evaluations of the magnitude of 1-year and maximum duration graft survival for different numbers of transfusions (1-5, 5-10, and ≥10 transfusions) versus no transfusions, respectively. In all analyses for 1-year (100.0 percent) and all analyses except one (95.5 percent) for maximum duration graft survival, a large benefit or small change was noted (Table 29). Thus, we concluded that different number of units of blood transfused has a beneficial to neutral effect on 1-year and maximum duration graft survival, and we graded the strength of the body of evidence for such effects to be low.

Higher number versus lower number of transfused units

Six and twelve analyses performed statistical evaluations to determine if higher versus lower number of transfused units had a significant effect on 1-year and maximum duration graft survival, respectively. For 1-year survival and maximum duration survival, all available analyses in the three different pairwise groups (≥5 versus 1-5, ≥10 versus 1-5, ≥10 versus 5-10) reported either a significant increase or no significant effect. None of the analyses found transfusion to have a significant negative impact on 1-year and maximum duration of graft survival (Table 30). Thus, we concluded that a higher number of units of transfused blood had a beneficial to neutral effect on 1-year and maximum duration graft survival, and we graded the strength of the body of evidence for such effects to be low.

Twelve and sixteen analyses performed evaluations of the magnitude of 1-year and maximum duration graft survival for higher versus lower number of blood transfusions, respectively. For 1-year survival, all available analyses in the three different pairwise groups (≥5 versus 1-5, >10 versus 1-5, >10 versus 5-10) reported either an increase or no effect on 1-year and maximum duration graft survival with a higher versus lower number of units infused. For maximum duration, in 15 of 16 analyses (93.8 percent), a beneficial or neutral effect was seen with higher versus lower number of transfusions (Table 30). Thus, we concluded that a higher number of units of transfused blood had a beneficial to neutral effect on 1-year and maximum duration graft survival, and we graded the strength of the body of evidence for such effects to be low.

Number of donors

No analysis reported results on 1-year and maximum duration graft survival. Therefore, there was insufficient data to grade the strength of evidence on the effect of number of donors on graft survival.

Patient Survival

Number of transfusions[37,73,142]

A total of 16 analyses, split evenly between those reporting 1-year (n=8) and those reporting maximum duration (n=8) patient survival, reported statistical results on the impact of different number of transfusions versus no transfusion. Regardless of the number of transfusions (1-5, 5-10, or ≥10 versus no transfusions), all analyses found no significant effect. As such, the conclusion was that there is a neutral effect on 1-year and maximum duration patient survival regardless of the number of transfusions versus receiving no transfusion. We graded the strength of evidence to be low (Table 31).

Similarly, all of the 14 analyses, split evenly between those reporting 1-year and those reporting maximum duration patient survival, reported statistical evaluations of the impact of higher transfusion intensities versus lower transfusion intensities. In every comparison of higher versus lower transfusion intensity, no significant effect on 1-year and maximum duration patient survival occurred. Thus, we concluded that number of transfusions did not have any significant impact on 1-year and maximum duration patient survival, and we graded the strength of the body of evidence for such effects to be low (Table 32).

Eight and seven analyses performed evaluations of the magnitude of different transfusion intensities (1-5, 5-10, or ≥10) compared to no transfusion on 1-year and maximum duration patient survival, respectively. All analyses found either a >10 percent increase or a small change within 10 percent in either direction in 1-year and maximum duration patient survival. We concluded that there was a large beneficial to neutral effect of different number of transfusions versus no transfusion on patient survival and we graded the strength of the body of evidence as low (Table 31).

Seven and five analyses evaluated the magnitude of higher transfusion intensities to lower transfusion intensities (≥5 vs. 1-5, >10 vs. 1-5, >10 vs. 5-10) on 1-year and maximum duration patient survival, respectively. All of the analyses reported a small change within 10 percent in either direction in survival on 1-year and maximum duration patient survival. We concluded that the number of transfusion has small impact on patient survival, and we graded the strength of the body of evidence for such effects to be low (Table 32).

Units of transfusions

No analysis reported results on 1-year and maximum duration patient survival. Thus, there was insufficient data to grade the strength of evidence on the effect of number of units of transfusions on patient survival.

Number of donors

No analysis reported results on 1-year and maximum duration patient survival. Therefore, there was insufficient data to grade the strength of evidence on the effect of number of donors on patient survival.

Multivariate Analysis Results

Seven analyses[138,151] evaluated the number of transfusions or the number of units transfused as a covariate in multivariate analysis assessing rejection. In five of these analyses, transfusion was a covariate but the remaining people in the dataset could include patients who received no transfusions (Table 33). In three of five (60.0 percent) of these analyses, the use of transfusions was an independent predictor of lesser rejection. Two other analyses specifically compared a higher intensity (>5 transfusions) to lower intensity of transfusions (1-5 transfusions) and lower intensity could not include no transfusions. One of the two analyses (50.0 percent) found that greater than five transfusions was an independent predictor of increasing the risk of rejection. Both of these latter analyses were from the same study and higher number of transfusions was significant for living donors (RR 1.29, p=0.003) but not for cadaver donors (1.02, P=0762).

Eighteen analyses[84,124,126,128,138,152-155] assessed the number of transfusions or the number of units transfused as a covariate in multivariate analysis evaluating graft survival. In six of the analyses (33.3 percent), transfusions of different intensities were independent predictors of worsening graft survival (Table 34). One analysis (6 percent) found that one or more transfusions were an independent predictor of benefiting graft survival. Eleven analyses (61.1 percent) did not find transfusions ranging from one to greater than 10 to be independent predictors of graft survival in either direction. When we evaluated only studies which explicitly compared a higher number of transfusions versus a lower number that could not include zero (no transfusions), 2 analyses were available and were both from the same study. In this study, the use of >5 transfusions was an independent predictor of worsening graft survival in both living and cadaver donors.

Seven analyses[124,128,154,156] evaluated the number of transfusions or the number of units transfused as a covariate in multivariate analysis assessing for patient survival (Table 35). Three of the analyses were from the same study.[138] In this study, the covariate "1-5 transfusions versus no transfusions" was not an independent predictor of patient survival. In this study, 1 analysis (14 percent) found that 6 to 10 transfusions versus no transfusion and another analysis (14 percent) found that >10 transfusions versus no transfusion were both independent predictors of worsening patient survival. One analysis (14 percent) from another trial found that transfusions greater than 40 units was a significant predictor of worsening patient survival. Four analyses (57 percent) determined that the number of transfusions or number of units transfused was not an independent predictor of patient survival in either direction but three of four of the analyses were limited to five or fewer transfusions.

In summary, transfusions were not an independent predictor of rejection, graft survival, or patient survival in either direction in a large number of analyses. Greater than five transfusions may have worsening graft and patient survival compared to one to five transfusions but the data are scant and may differ based on whether the graft is from a living or cadaver donor.

Table 25. Insight into body of literature: Number/Units of transfusions and number of donors (KQ1bii)

	Rejection	Graft Survival	Patient sSurvival	Validity of Studies
KQ 1bii. Number/Units of Transfusion, Number of Donors	CCT 1 Analysis POBS None ROBS 18 Analyses	CCT 1-year –9 Analyses Max time –11 Analyses POBS 1-year –6 Analyses Max time – 9 Analyses ROBS 1-year –112 Analyses Max time –118 Analyses	CCT None POBS None ROBS 1-year –15 Analyses Max time –15 Analyses	Good 0 study Fair 7 studies Poor 30 studies

CCT=clinical controlled trial, KQ=key question, Max=maximum followup time, POBS=prospective observational studies, ROBS=retrospective observational studies,

Table 26. Impact of any number/unit of transfusions, or number of donors on rejection (KQ1bii)

KQ 1bii Graft Rejection Any Time Point	Significant Decreases in Rejection	No Significant Effect on Rejection	Significant Increases in Rejection	Decreased Risk of Rejection *	No Change in Rejection †	Increased Risk of Rejection *
Number of transfusions‡	2/5 (40.0%)	3/5 (60.0%)	0/5 (0.0%)	6/18 (33.3%)	10/18 (55.6%)	2/18 (11.1%)
Number of units of transfusion‡	0/1 (0.0%)	1/1 (100.0%)	0/1 (0.0%)	0/1 (0.0%)	1/1 (100.0%)	0/1 (0.0%)

| Number of donors | No data | No data | No data | No data | No data | No data |

*Data either showing a decrease/increase of any magnitude or notation in text stating a decrease/increase
†Data either showing no difference, or notation in text stating no change
‡Any number/units of transfusions versus any other number/units of transfusions

Table 27. Impact of number of transfusions on graft survival: *intensity of transfusion versus no transfusion* (KQ1bii)

Number of transfusions	Significant Increases in Survival	No Significant Effect	Significant Decreases in Survival	>10% Increase in Survival	10% to -10% Change in Survival	>10% Decrease in Survival
1-5 versus 0						
1-Year graft survival	1/5 (20.0%)	4/5 (80.0%)	0/5 (0.0%)	10/19 (52.6%)	9/19 (47.4%)	0/19 (0.0%)
Max duration graft survival	2/4 (50.0%)	2/4 (50.0%)	0/4 (0.0%)	9/20 (45.0%)	10/20 (50.0%)	1/20 (5.0%)
5-10/>5 versus 0						
1-Year graft survival	2/4 (50.0%)	1/4 (25.0%)	1/4 (25.0%)	11/20 (55.0%)	7/20 (35.0%)	2/20 (10.0%)
Max duration graft survival	2/4 (50.0%)	0/4 (0.0%)	2/4 (50.0%)	10/21 (47.6%)	8/21 (38.1%)	3/21 (14.3%)
≥10 versus 0						
1-Year graft survival	1/3 (33.3%)	2/3 (66.7%)	0/3 (0.0%)	9/12 (75.0%)	3/12 (25.0%)	0/12 (0.0%)
Max duration graft survival	1/1 (100.0%)	0/1 (0.0%)	0/1 (0.0%)	9/12 (75.0%)	3/12 (25.0%)	0/12 (0.0%)

Table 28. Impact of number of transfusions on graft survival: *higher versus lower number of transfusions* (KQ1bii)

Number of transfusions	Significant Increases in Survival	No Significant Effect	Significant Decreases in Survival	>10% Increase in Survival	10% to -10% Change in Survival	>10% Decrease in Survival
5-10/>5 versus 1-5						
1-Year graft survival	4/7 (57.1%)	1/7 (14.3%)	2/7 (28.6%)	9/21 (42.9%)	12/21 (57.1%)	0/21 (0.0%)
Max duration graft survival	6/11 (54.5%)	1/11 (9.1%)	4/11 (36.4%)	11/28 (39.3%)	11/28 (39.3%)	6/28 (21.4%)
≥10 versus 1-5						

Number of transfusions	Significant Increases in Survival	No Significant Effect	Significant Decreases in Survival	>10% Increase in Survival	10% to -10% Change in Survival	>10% Decrease in Survival
1-Year graft survival	0/2 (0.0%)	2/2 (100.0%)	0/2 (0.0%)	4/10 (40.0%)	6/10 (60.0%)	0/10 (0.0%)
Max duration graft survival	No data	No data	No data	3/9 (33.3%)	6/9 (66.7%)	0/9 (0.0%)
≥10 versus 5-10						
1-Year graft survival	0/2 (0.0%)	2/2 (100.0%)	0/2 (0.0%)	2/12 (16.7%)	10/12 (83.3%)	0/12 (0.0%)
Max duration graft survival	No data	No data	No data	1/11 (9.1%)	10/11 (90.9%)	0/11 (0.0%)

Table 29. Impact of units of blood on graft survival: *increasing number of units versus no transfusion* (KQ1bii)

KQ 1bii Units of blood	Significant Increases in Survival	No Significant Effect	Significant Decreases in Survival	>10% Increase in Survival	10% to -10% Change in Survival	>10% Decrease in Survival
1-5 versus 0						
1-Year graft survival	1/5 (20.0%)	4/5 (80.0%)	0/5 (0.0%)	4/10 (40.0%)	6/10 (60.0%)	0/10 (0.0%)
Max duration graft survival	2/7 (28.6%)	5/7 (71.4%)	0/7 (0.0%)	5/10 (50.0%)	4/10 (40.0%)	1/10 (10.0%)
5-10/ >5 versus 0						
1-Year graft survival	1/4 (25.0%)	3/4 (75.0%)	0/4 (0.0%)	3/8 (37.5%)	5/8 (62.5%)	0/8 (0.0%)
Max duration graft survival	2/5 (40.0%)	3/5 (60.0%)	0/5 (0.0%)	5/9 (55.6%)	3/9 (33.3%)	1/9 (11.1%)
≥10 versus 0						
1-Year graft survival	1/2 (50.0%)	1/2 (50.0%)	0/2 (0.0%)	3/3 (100.0%)	0/3 (0.0%)	0/3 (0.0%)
Max duration graft survival	2/4 (50.0%)	2/4 (50.0%)	0/4 (0.0%)	2/3 (66.7%)	1/3 (33.3%)	0/3 (0.0%)

Table 30. Impact of units of blood on graft survival: *greater number of units versus lower numbers of units* (KQ1bii)

KQ 1bii Units of blood	Significant Increases in Survival	No Significant Effect	Significant Decreases in Survival	>10% Increase in Survival	10% to -10% Change in Survival	>10% Decrease in Survival

KQ 1bii Units of blood	Significant Increases in Survival	No Significant Effect	Significant Decreases in Survival	>10% Increase in Survival	10% to -10% Change in Survival	>10% Decrease in Survival
5-10/ >5 versus 1-5						
1-Year graft survival	0/4 (0.0%)	4/4 (100.0%)	0/4 (0.0%)	1/8 (12.5%)	7/8 (87.5%)	0/8 (0.0%)
Max duration graft survival	0/7 (0.0%)	7/7 (100.0%)	0/7 (0.0%)	1/11 (9.1%)	9/11 (81.8%)	1/11 (9.1%)
≥10 versus 1-5						
1-Year graft survival	0/1 (0.0%)	1/1 (100.0%)	0/1 (0.0%)	1/3 (33.3%)	2/3 (66.7%)	0/3 (0.0%)
Max duration graft survival	0/3 (0.0%)	3/3 (100.0%)	0/3 (0.0%)	1/3 (33.3%)	2/3 (66.7%)	0/3 (0.0%)
≥10 versus 5-10						
1-Year graft survival	0/1 (0.0%)	1/1 (100.0%)	0/1 (0.0%)	0/1 (0.0%)	1/1 (100.0%)	0/1 (0.0%)
Max duration graft survival	0/2 (0.0%)	2/2 (100.0%)	0/2 (0.0%)	1/2 (50.0%)	1/2 (50.0%)	0/2 (0.0%)

Table 31. Impact of number of transfusions on patient survival: *intensity of transfusion versus no transfusion* (KQ1bii)

Number of transfusions	Significant Increases in Survival	No Significant Effect	Significant Decreases in Survival	>10% Increase in Survival	10% to -10% Change in Survival	>10% Decrease in Survival
1-5 versus 0						
1-Year patient survival	0/3 (0.0%)	3/3 (100.0%)	0/3 (0.0%)	0/3 (0.0%)	3/3 (100.0%)	0/3 (0.0%)
Max duration patient survival	0/3 (0.0%)	3/3 (100.0%)	0/3 (0.0%)	0/3 (0.0%)	3/3 (100.0%)	0/3 (0.0%)
5-10/ >5 versus 0						
1-Year patient survival	0/3 (0.0%)	3/3 (100.0%)	0/3 (0.0%)	1/3 (33.3%)	2/3 (66.7%)	0/3 (0.0%)
Max duration patient survival	0/3 (0.0%)	3/3 (100.0%)	0/3 (0.0%)	1/3 (33.3%)	2/3 (66.7%)	0/3 (0.0%)
≥10 versus 0						
1-Year patient survival	0/2 (0.0%)	2/2 (100.0%)	0/2 (0.0%)	1/2 (50.0%)	1/2 (50.0%)	0/2 (0.0%)

Number of transfusions	Significant Increases in Survival	No Significant Effect	Significant Decreases in Survival	>10% Increase in Survival	10% to -10% Change in Survival	>10% Decrease in Survival
Max duration patient survival	0/2 (0.0%)	2/2 (100.0%)	0/2 (0.0%)	0/1 (0.0%)	1/1 (100.0%)	0/1 (0.0%)

Table 32. Impact of number of transfusions on patient survival: *higher versus lower number of transfusions* (KQ1bii)

Number of transfusions	Significant Increases in Survival	No Significant Effect	Significant Decreases in Survival	>10% Increase in Survival	10% to -10% Change in Survival	>10% Decrease in Survival
5-10/ >5 versus 1-5						
1-Year patient survival	0/3 (0.0%)	3/3 (100.0%)	0/3 (0.0%)	0/3 (0.0%)	3/3 (100.0%)	0/3 (0.0%)
Max duration patient survival	0/3 (0.0%)	3/3 (100.0%)	0/3 (0.0%)	0/3 (0.0%)	3/3 (100.0%)	0/3 (0.0%)
≥10 versus 1-5						
1-Year patient survival	0/2 (0.0%)	2/2 (100.0%)	0/2 (0.0%)	0/2 (0.0%)	2/2 (100.0%)	0/2 (0.0%)
Max duration patient survival	0/2 (0.0%)	2/2 (100.0%)	0/2 (0.0%)	0/1 (0.0%)	1/1 (100.0%)	0/1 (0.0%)
≥10 versus 5-10						
1-Year patient survival	0/2 (0.0%)	2/2 (100.0%)	0/2 (0.0%)	0/2 (0.0%)	2/2 (100.0%)	0/2 (0.0%)
Max duration patient survival	0/2 (0.0%)	2/2 (100.0%)	0/2 (0.0%)	0/1 (0.0%)	1/1 (100.0%)	0/1 (0.0%)

Table 33. Multivariate results: Impact of number/units of transfusion on rejection (KQ1bii)

Study, Year Total N	Analysis Type	Covariate	Outcome Evaluated	Multivariate Results	Significant Effect
Higgins RM, 2004 N=265	Multiple logistic regression	3 or more transfused blood units before transplant	Acute rejection	OR 0.49 (0.29-0.83), P=0.008	Transfusion benefits rejection
Chavers BM, 1997 LD* N=2007	NR	1-5 transfusions vs. 0	First acute rejection episode	RR 0.86, P=0.036	Transfusion benefits rejection
Chavers BM, 1997 CAD† N=2008	NR	1-5 transfusions vs. 0	First acute rejection episode	RR 0.86, P=0.046	Transfusion benefits rejection

Study, Year Total N	Analysis Type	Covariate	Outcome Evaluated	Multivariate Results	Significant Effect
Chavers BM, 1997 LD* N=2007	NR	>5 transfusions vs. 0	First acute rejection episode	RR 1.11, P=0.284	NA
Chavers BM, 1997 CAD† N=2008	NR	>5 transfusions vs. 0	First acute rejection episode	RR 0.88, P=0.123	NA
Chavers BM, 1997 LD* N=2007	NR	>5 transfusions vs. 1-5	First acute rejection episode	RR 1.29, P=0.003	>5 transfusions worsens rejection
Chavers BM, 1997 CAD† N=2008	NR	>5 transfusions vs. 1-5	First acute rejection episode	RR 1.02, P=0.762	NA

* A separate analysis involving patients receiving living-donor renal transplants
† A separate analysis involving patients receiving cadaver renal transplants
CAD=cadaver transplants; LD=living donor; N=number of patients in analysis; NR=not reported; NS=not significant; OR=odds ratio; RR=relative risk

Table 34. Multivariate results: Impact of number/units of transfusion on graft survival (KQ1bii)

Study, Year Total N	Analysis Type	Covariate	Outcome Evaluated	Multivariate Results	Significant Effect
Tang H, 2008 N=2882	Cox*	1-5 pre-transplant transfusions vs. 0	Graft survival	HR 1.21 (0.95-1.54), P=0.124	NA
Tang H, 2008 N=2882	Cox*	6-10 pre-transplant transfusions vs. 0	Graft survival	HR 1.10 (0.72-1.69), P=0.652	NA
Tang H, 2008 N=2882	Cox*	>10 pre-transplant transfusions vs. 0	Graft survival	HR 1.10 (0.73-1.69), P=0.625	NA
Park YH, 2004 N=77	Cox*	Preoperative multiple transfusion history	Graft loss	RR 4.2, P=NR	NA
Bunnapradist S, 2003 N=7079	Cox*	1-5 pretransplant blood transfusions	Graft failure	HR 1.27 (1.07-1.49), P=0.005	Transfusion worsens graft survival
Agarwal SK, 2002 N=144	NR	Number of blood transfusions	Graft survival	NR, P=NS	NA
Montagnino G, 2000 N=143	Cox*	Blood transfusions (0 vs. ≥ 1)	Graft survival	RR 1.99 (1.021-3.889), P=0.043	Transfusion benefits graft survival

Study, Year Total N	Analysis Type	Covariate	Outcome Evaluated	Multivariate Results	Significant Effect
Chavers BM, 1997 LD† N=2007	NR	1-5 transfusions vs. 0	Graft failure	RR 1.04, P=0.770	NA
Chavers BM, 1997 CAD‡ N=2008	NR	1-5 transfusions vs. 0	Graft failure	RR 0.85, P=0.200	NA
Chavers BM, 1997 LD† N=2007	NR	>5 transfusions vs. 0	Graft failure	RR 1.64, P=0.002	Transfusion worsens graft survival
Chavers BM, 1997 CAD‡ N=2008	NR	>5 transfusions vs. 0	Graft failure	RR 1.15, P=0.288	NA
Chavers BM, 1997 LD† N=2007	NR	>5 transfusions vs. 1-5	Graft failure	RR 1.58, P=0.001	>5 transfusions worsen graft survival
Chavers BM, 1997 CAD‡ N=2008	NR	>5 transfusions vs. 1-5	Graft failure	RR 1.35, P=0.002	>5 transfusions worsen graft survival
Poli F, 1995 N=416	Cox*	Pre-transplant transfusion (0 vs. >0)	Graft survival	RR 1.2 (0.7-2.1), P=0.4	NA
Sautner T, 1994 N=146	Stepwise logistic regression	Number of pretransplant transfusions (5-10)	Graft loss	RR 1.7, P=0.02	Transfusion worsens graft survival
Sautner T, 1994 N=146	Stepwise logistic regression	Number of pretransplant transfusions (>10)	Graft loss	RR 6-fold increase, P=0.02	Transfusion worsens graft survival
CMTSG, 1986 CyA§ N=142	Cox*	Transfusion< 4 units N=67 (47%)	Graft loss	RR 0.99, P=NS	NA
CMTSG, 1986 Control‖ N=149	Cox*	Transfusion< 4 units N=75 (50%)	Graft loss	RR 1.35, P=NS	NA

* Cox proportional hazards regression analysis
† A separate analysis involving patients receiving living-donor renal transplants
‡ A separate analysis involving patients receiving cadaver renal transplants
§ Patients received immunosuppression with cyclosporine
‖ Patients received control immunosuppression with azathioprine

CAD=cadaver transplants; CMTSG=Canadian Multicenter Transplant Study Group; CyA=cyclosporine; HR=hazard ratio; LD=living donor; N=number of patients in analysis; NR=not reported; NS=not significant; RR=relative risk

Table 35. Multivariate results: Impact of number/units of transfusion on patient survival (KQ1bii)

Study, Year Total N	Analysis Type	Covariate	Outcome Evaluated	Multivariate Results	Significant Effect
Tang H, 2008 N=2882	Cox*	1-5 pre-transplant transfusions vs. 0	Patient death	HR 1.29 (0.97-1.72), P=0.083	NA
Tang H, 2008 N=2882	Cox*	6-10 pre-transplant transfusions vs. 0	Patient death	HR 1.64 (1.04-2.58), P<0.05	Transfusion worsens patient survival
Tang H, 2008 N=2882	Cox*	>10 pre-transplant transfusions vs. 0	Patient death	HR 1.98 (1.28-3.05), P<0.005	Transfusion worsens patient survival
Herget-Rosenthal S, 2003 N=40	Stepwise logistic regression	Multiple transfusions greater than 40 units	Patient death	RR 3.1 (1.1-9.2), P=0.03	Transfusion worsens patient survival
Agarwal SK, 2002 N=144	NR	Number of blood transfusions	Patient survival	NR, P=NS	NA
CMTSG, 1986 CyA† N=142	Cox*	Transfusion< 4 units	Patient death	RR 0.86, P=NS	NA
CMTSG, 1986 Control‡ N=149	Cox*	Transfusion< 4 units	Patient death	RR 0.98, P=NS	NA

* Cox proportional hazards regression analysis
† Patients received immunosuppression with cyclosporine
‡ Patients received control immunosuppression with azathioprine
CMTSG=Canadian Multicenter Transplant Study Group; CyA=cyclosporine; HR=hazard ratio; N=number of patients in analysis; NR=not reported; NS=not significant; RR=relative risk

Key Question 1biii. Is any such impact of red blood cell transfusions on renal transplant outcomes altered by the use of leukocyte-depleted blood?

Four unique studies were included in the evaluation of the use of leukocyte-depleted blood on renal transplant outcomes.[77,83,157,158] One of the studies was a controlled clinical trial, two were prospective observational studies and one was a retrospective observational study. Two studies (50 percent) were rated as fair quality, and two studies (50 percent) were rated as poor quality. Of the 12 analyses reported in these studies, 16.7 percent were from the controlled clinical trial, 66.6 percent were from the prospective observational study, and 16.7 percent were from the retrospective observational study. None (0 percent), 10 (83.3 percent), and 2 (16.7 percent) included results for graft rejection, graft survival and patient survival, respectively (Table 36).

Rejection

None of the included analyses evaluated the impact of leukocyte-depleted blood transfusions on rejection (Table 37). Thus, we concluded that the strength of the body of evidence was insufficient upon which to base any conclusion.

Graft Survival

Leukocyte-depleted versus no transfusion

None of the included analyses evaluated the significant effects of leukocyte-depleted blood versus no transfusion on 1-year or maximum duration graft survival (Table 38). To be considered in this evaluation, studies had to provide a p-value, 95 percent confidence interval, or explicitly state whether or not statistical significance was achieved. As a result, we found that the body of evidence was insufficient.

Two analyses found the magnitude of effect of leukocyte-depleted transfusions versus no transfusion was greater than a 10 percent increase on 1-year and maximum duration graft survival.[77,83] We concluded that the use of leukocyte-depleted blood versus no transfusion may have beneficial effect on 1-year and maximum duration graft survival, and that the strength of evidence for these effects was low.

Leukocyte-depleted versus therapeutic transfusion

One study evaluated the significant effects of leukocyte-depleted transfusions versus therapeutic transfusions, and reported no significant effect on 1-year and maximum duration graft survival.[77] Leukocyte-depleted blood was not found to significantly increase or decrease graft survival (Table 39). Thus, leukocyte-depleted transfusions versus therapeutic transfusions may have a neutral effect on 1-year and maximum duration graft survival, but the strength of evidence was insufficient.

Two analyses found the magnitude of effect of leukocyte-depleted blood versus therapeutic transfusions to be a small change within 10 percent in either direction in survival with regard to 1-year graft survival.[77,157] For maximum duration graft survival, one analysis found the magnitude of effect to be greater than 10 percent,[77] and one analysis found the magnitude of effect to be a small change within 10 percent in either direction.[157] We concluded that the use of leukocyte-depleted transfusions versus therapeutic transfusions may have a neutral to beneficial effect on 1-year and maximum duration graft survival, and that the strength of evidence for these effects was low.

One study examined the effects of leukocyte-depleted blood versus leukocyte-free blood and evaluated only the magnitude of effect on 1-year and maximum duration graft survival.[158] For both 1-year and maximum duration graft survival, the use of leukocyte-depleted blood versus leukocyte-free blood resulted in a greater than 10 percent increase in graft survival. This study does not explicitly meet the requirement to answer this question.

Patient Survival

Leukocyte-depleted versus no transfusion

None of the included analyses evaluated the significant effects of leukocyte-depleted blood versus no transfusion on 1-year patient survival (Table 38). One analysis determined that the use of leukocyte-depleted transfusion versus no transfusion had no significant effect on the maximum duration of patient survival.[77] This analysis did not find that the use of leukocyte-depleted blood versus no transfusion resulted in a significant increase or decrease in maximum duration patient survival. As only one analysis provided evidence, we concluded that the strength of evidence was insufficient to determine any conclusion.

None of the included analyses determined the magnitude of effect of leukocyte-depleted blood versus no transfusion on 1-year patient survival. One analysis found that the use of leukocyte-depleted blood versus therapeutic transfusion had a greater than 10 percent increase in patient survival.[77] We found that the strength of evidence was insufficient to determine a conclusion.

Leukocyte-depleted versus therapeutic transfusion

None of the included analyses evaluated the significant effects of leukocyte-depleted blood versus therapeutic transfusions on 1-year patient survival. One analysis determined that the use of leukocyte-depleted transfusion versus therapeutic transfusions had no significant effect on the maximum duration of patient survival.[77] This analysis did not find that the use of leukocyte-depleted blood resulted in a significant increase or decrease in maximum duration patient survival (Table 39). As only one analysis provided evidence, we concluded that the strength of evidence was insufficient to determine any conclusion.

None of the included analyses determined the magnitude of effect of leukocyte-depleted transfusions versus therapeutic transfusions on 1-year patient survival. One analysis found that the use of leukocyte-depleted blood versus no transfusion had a greater than 10 percent increase in patient survival.[77] We found that the strength of evidence was insufficient to determine a conclusion.

Table 36. Insight into body of literature: Leukocyte-depleted blood (KQ 1biii)

	Rejection	Graft Survival	Patient survival	Validity of Studies
KQ 1biii. Leukocyte-depleted blood	CCT None POBS None ROBS None	CCT 1-year – 1 analysis Max time – 1 analysis POBS 1-year – 2 Analyses Max time – 2 Analyses ROBS 1-year – 1 Analysis Max time – 1 Analysis	CCT None POBS 1-year – None Max time – 2 analyses ROBS None	Good None Fair 2 studies Poor 2 studies

CCT=clinical controlled trial, KQ=key question, Max=maximum followup time, POBS=prospective observational studies, ROBS=retrospective observational studies

Table 37. Impact of leukocyte-depleted transfusions versus no or therapeutic transfusion on rejection (KQ 1biii)

KQ 1biii	Significant Decreases in Rejection	No Significant Effect on Rejection	Significant Increases in Rejection	Decreased Risk of Rejection*	No Change in Rejection†	Increased Risk of Rejection*
Graft Rejection Any Time Point	No data	No data	No data	No data	No data	No data

*Data either showing a decrease/increase of any magnitude or notation in text stating a decrease/increase
†Data either showing no difference, or notation in text stating no change

Table 38. Impact of leukocyte-depleted transfusions versus no transfusion on graft and patient survival (KQ 1biii)

KQ 1biii	Significant Increases in Survival	No Significant Effect	Significant Decreases in Survival	>10% Increase in Survival	10% to -10% Change in Survival	>10% Decrease in Survival
1-Year Graft Survival	No data	No data	No data	2/2 (100.0%)	0/2 (0.0%)	0/2 (0.0%)
Max Duration Graft Survival	No data	No data	No data	2/2 (100.0%)	0/2 (0.0%)	0/2 (0.0%)
1-Year Patient Survival	No data	No data	No data	No data	No data	No data
Max Duration Patient Survival	0/1 (0.0%)	1/1 (100.0%)	0/1 (0.0%)	0/1 (0.0%)	1/1 (100.0%)	0/1 (0.0%)

Table 39. Impact of leukocyte-depleted transfusions versus therapeutic transfusions on graft and patient survival (KQ 1biii)

KQ 1biii	Significant Increases in Survival	No Significant Effect	Significant Decreases in Survival	>10% Increase in Survival	10% to -10% Change in Survival	>10% Decrease in Survival
1-Year Graft Survival	0/1 (0.0%)	1/1 (100.0%)	0/1 (0.0%)	0/2 (0.0%)	2/2 (100.0%)	0/2 (0.0%)
Max Duration Graft Survival	0/1 (0.0%)	1/1 (100.0%)	0/1 (0.0%)	1/2 (50.0%)	1/2 (50.0%)	0/2 (0.0%)
1-Year Patient Survival	No data	No data	No data	No data	No data	No data
Max Duration Patient Survival	0/1 (0.0%)	1/1 (100.0%)	0/1 (0.0%)	1/1 (100.0%)	0/1 (0.0%)	0/1 (0.0%)

Key Question 1biv-v. Is any such impact of red blood cell transfusions on renal transplant outcomes altered by changes in immunosuppression regimens (pre-cyclosporine, cyclosporine, later multi-drug regimens) or other changes in management over time?

We answered these two key questions together. The time period before 1984 denoted the pre-cyclosporine era, 1984-1991 denoted the cyclosporine era, and 1992-present denoted the era of newer multidrug regimens. Doing the analysis via time periods also allowed the changes in organ procurement, preservation, and transplantation as well as other management changes occurring over these time periods to be reflected in the evaluations.

Ninety-two unique studies were included in the evaluation of the impact of transfusions from before 1984,[20,24-27,29,31-36,39-45,47-64,66,67,69,70,72-76,78-83,85,86,88-93,98-103,105-108,110,111,114-117,119,120] 1984-1991,[17,23,37,38,65,71,84,112] and 1992 to present,[14-16,18,19,113] of which a majority of the studies (84.8 percent) evaluated the effect of transfusion on renal allograft outcomes before 1984, while 8.7 percent and 6.5 percent reported such effects during 1984 to 1991 and from 1992 to present, respectively. Sixty-eight (87.2 percent) of the 78 studies (conducted before 1984) were retrospective observational studies. 8 (10.2 percent) were prospective studies, and only two were controlled trials (2.6 percent). Over ninety percent of the studies conducted during this time period were rated as poor. Eight studies (rated as 1 good, 3 fair, and 4 poor quality) that evaluated transfusion effects during 1984 to 1992, were retrospective studies and controlled trials, respectively. For the four (66.7 percent) rated as good, and two fair (33.3 percent) quality studies that were conducted after 1992 to present, four (66.7 percent) were clinical trials and two (33.3 percent) were retrospective studies (Table 40).

Rejection[20,35,42,44,47,50,69,70,73,76,89,92,98,102,103,108]

Seven, two, and two analyses evaluated the time periods before 1984, 1984–1991, and 1992–present, respectively. Five of seven (71.4 percent), two of two (100.0 percent), and one of two (50.0 percent) analyses found a significant decrease in rejection with the use of transfusion from before 1984, 1984-1991, and 1992-present, respectively (Table 41). The remainder of the analyses found significant increases in rejection with the use of transfusion over these time periods. So while the number of analyses in the time period 1992-present was very small, it appears some measure of the protective effect of transfusion in earlier time periods was lost with 50 percent of analyses showing a benefit and 50 percent showing a detriment with transfusion. The conclusion was that up to the year 1992, transfusion has a beneficial to neutral effect on rejection, but that after 1992 transfusion may or may not provide this effect. We graded the strength of the body of evidence for such effects to be low.

Nineteen, seven, and nine analyses evaluated the directional change in rejection associated with transfusion use. Fifteen of nineteen (78.9 percent), five of seven (71.4 percent), and three of nine (33.3 percent) analyses found a decrease in rejection from before 1984, 1984–1991, and 1992-present, respectively (Table 41). As the number of analyses finding a decrease in rejection went down from time periods before 1992 to the

1992–present, the number of analyses showing an increase in rejection increased from 3 of 19 (15.8 percent) and one of seven (14.3 percent) over the time periods before 1984 and 1984–1991 to 4 of 9 (44.5 percent) analyses in the time period from 1992 to the present. Like for the evaluation above looking at statistical significance, in the time period 1992-present it appears some measure of the protective effect of transfusion was lost, although a majority of analyses (55.5 percent) still found either a beneficial or neutral effect on rejection. The conclusion was that up to the year 1992, transfusion has a beneficial to neutral effect on rejection, but that after 1992 transfusion may or may not provide this effect. We graded the strength of the body of evidence for such effects to be low.

Graft Survival[20,24-27,29,31-36,39-45,47-64,66,67,70,72-83,85,86,88,90-93,98-103,105-108,110,111,114-117,119,120]

We evaluated for significant 1-year and maximum duration graft survival with the use of transfusion over the time periods before 1984 (40 and 49 analyses), 1984–1991 (4 and 6 analyses), and 1992-present (3 and 2 analyses), respectively (Table 42). For 1-year and for maximum duration graft survival, for each time period evaluated all of the analyses found either a significant increase or no significant impact on graft survival associated with the use transfusion. No analysis found a significant decrease in graft survival. However, there was shift from most analyses showing a beneficial effect to a no significant effect over time. The conclusion was that regardless of the time period, transfusion has either a beneficial or neutral effect on graft survival with a shifting away from beneficial to solidly neutral in more contemporary practice. We graded the strength of the body of evidence for such effects to be low.

We evaluated for a greater than 10 percent increase or decrease or a less dramatic change (10 percent to -10 percent) on 1-year and maximum duration graft survival with the use of transfusion over the time periods before 1984 (93 and 102 analyses), 1984-1991 (6 and 8 analyses), and 1992-present (nine and nine analyses), respectively (Table 42). For 1-year and for maximum duration graft survival, for each time period evaluated a vast majority (96-100 percent) of the analyses found either a >10 percent increase or a small change within 10 percent in either direction on graft survival associated with the use transfusion. However, there was shift towards more analyses showing a small magnitude of change on graft survival over time. The conclusion was that regardless of the time period, transfusion has a beneficial to neutral effect on graft survival. We graded the strength of the body of evidence to be low.

Patient Survival[29,33,50,53,59,62,77,86,88,89,93,99,103,106,108,111,114,120]

We evaluated for significant 1-year and maximum duration patient survival with the use of transfusion over the time periods before 1984 (9 and 12 analyses), 1984-1991 (5 and 5 analyses), and 1992-present (3 and 1 analyses), respectively (Table 42). For 1-year and for maximum duration patient survival, for each time period evaluated all of the analyses found either a significant increase or no significant impact on patient survival associated with the use transfusion. The predominant number of analyses found no significant effect over time and no analysis found a significant decrease in patient survival. The conclusion was that regardless of the time period, transfusion has a beneficial to neutral effect on patient survival. We graded the strength of the body of evidence for such effects to be low.

We evaluated for a greater than 10 percent increase or decrease or a less dramatic change (10 percent to -10 percent) on 1-year and maximum duration patient survival with the use of transfusion over the time periods before 1984 (19 and 23 analyses), 1984–1991 (5 and 8 analyses), and 1992-present (6 and 6 analyses), respectively (Table 42). For 1-year and for maximum duration patient survival, for each time period evaluated a vast majority (87-100 percent) of the analyses found either a >10 percent increase or a small change within 10 percent in either direction on patient survival associated with the use transfusion. The predominant number of analyses found no significant effect over time. The conclusion was that regardless of the time period, transfusion has a beneficial to neutral effect on patient survival. We graded the strength of the body of evidence to be low.

Table 40. Insight into body of literature: Impact of transfusions over different time periods (KQ 1biv-v)

KQ 1b(iv-v)	Rejection	Graft Survival	Patient survival	Validity of Studies
Before 1984	CCT 1 Analyses POBS None ROBS 18 Analyses	CCT 1-Year – 3 Analyses Max Time – 3 Analyses POBS 1-Year – 11 Analyses Max Time – 14 Analyses ROBS 1-Year – 79 Analyses Max Time – 85 Analyses	CCT None POBS 1-Year – 1 Analyses Max Time – 3 Analyses ROBS 1-Year – 18 Analyses Max Time – 20 Analyses	Good None Fair 5 studies Poor 73 studies
Initiated 1984-1992	CCT 2 Analyses POBS None ROBS 5 Analyses	CCT 1-Year – 2 Analyses Max Time – 2 Analyses POBS None ROBS 1-Year – 4 Analyses Max Time –6 Analyses	CCT 1-Year – 2 Analyses Max Time – 2 Analyses POBS None ROBS 1-Year – 3 Analyses Max Time – 5 Analyses	Good 1 study Fair 3 studies Poor 4 studies
1992-Present	CCT 5 Analyses POBS None ROBS 4 Analyses	CCT 1-Year – 5 Analyses Max Time – 5 Analyses POBS None ROBS 1-Year – 4 Analyses Max Time – 4 Analyses	CCT 1-Year – 5 Analyses Max Time – 5 Analyses POBS None ROBS 1-Year – 1 Analyses Max Time – 1 Analyses	Good 4 studies Fair 2 studies Poor 0 study

CCT=clinical controlled trial, KQ=key question, Max=maximum followup time, POBS=prospective observational studies, ROBS=retrospective observational studies

Table 41. Impact of transfusion over different time periods on rejection (KQ1biv-v)

Impact of transfusions on graft rejection	Significant Decreases in Rejection	No Significant Effect on Rejection	Significant Increases in Rejection	Decrease Risk of Rejection*	No Change in Rejection†	Increase Risk of Rejection*
Before 1984	5/7 (71.4%)	0/7 (0.0%)	2/7 (28.6%)	15/19 (78.9%)	1/19 (5.3%)	3/19 (15.8%)
Initiated 1984 to 1991	2/2 (100.0%)	0/2 (0.0%)	0/2 (0.0%)	5/7 (71.4%)	1/7 (14.3%)	1/7 (14.3%)
1992 – Present	1/2 (50.0%)	0/2 (0.0%)	1/2 (50.0%)	3/9 (33.3%)	2/9 (22.2%)	4/9 (44.5%)

*Data either showing a decrease/increase of any magnitude or notation in text stating a decrease/increase
†Data either showing no difference, or notation in text stating no change

Table 42. Impact of transfusions over different time periods on graft and patient survival (KQ 1biv-v)

Impact of transfusions on:	Significant Increases in Survival	No Significant Effect	Significant Decreases in Survival	>10% Increase in Survival	10% to -10% Change in Survival	>10% Decrease in Survival
1 Year Graft Survival						
Before 1984	24/40 (60.0%)	16/40 (40.0%)	0/40 (0.0%)	60/93 (64.5%)	30/93 (32.3%)	3/93 (3.2%)
Initiated 1984 to 1991	0/4 (0.0%)	4/4 (100.0%)	0/4 (0.0%)	1/6 (16.7%)	5/6 (83.3%)	0/6 (0.0%)
1992 – Present	0/3 (0.0%)	3/3 (100.0%)	0/3 (0.0%)	1/9 (11.1%)	8/9 (88.9%)	0/9 (0.0%)
Max Time Graft Survival						
Before 1984	23/49 (46.9%)	26/49 (53.1%)	0/49 (0.0%)	65/102 (63.7%)	33/102 (32.4%)	4/102 (3.9%)
Initiated 1984 to 1991	2/6 (33.3%)	4/6 (66.7%)	0/6 (0.0%)	3/8 (37.5%)	5/8 (62.5%)	0/8 (0.0%)
1992 – Present	0/2 (0.0%)	2/2 (100.0%)	0/2 (0.0%)	2/9 (22.2%)	7/9 (77.7%)	0/9 (0.0%)
1 Year Patient Survival						
Before 1984	0/9 (0.0%)	9/9 (100.0%)	0/9 (0.0%)	1/19 (5.3%)	16/19 (84.2%)	2/19 (10.5%)
Initiated 1984 to 1991	0/5 (0.0%)	5/5 (100.0%)	0/5 (0.0%)	0/5 (0.0%)	5/5 (100.0%)	0/5 (0.0%)
1992 – Present	0/3 (0.0%)	3/3 (100.0%)	0/3 (0.0%)	0/6 (0.0%)	6/6 (100.0%)	0/6 (0.0%)

Impact of transfusions on:	Significant Increases in Survival	No Significant Effect	Significant Decreases in Survival	>10% Increase in Survival	10% to -10% Change in Survival	>10% Decrease in Survival
Max Time Patient Survival						
Before 1984	1/12 (8.3%)	11/12 (91.7%)	0/12 (0.0%)	6/23 (26.1%)	14/23 (60.9%)	3/23 (13.0%)
Initiated 1984 to 1991	0/5 (0.0%)	5/5 (100.0%)	0/5 (0.0%)	2/8 (25%)	5/8 (62.5%)	1/8 (12.5%)
1992 – Present	0/1 (0.0%)	1/1 (100.0%)	0/1 (0.0%)	0/6 (0.0%)	6/6 (100.0%)	0/6 (0.0%)

Key Question 2a. How have panel reactive antibody (PRA) assays changed over time? Do all PRA assays measure the same things? What things contribute to intra-assay variability (e.g., time, when during the dialysis cycle the sample was obtained, statin use)? How correlative or independent of one another are these measures?

Panel Reactive Antibody Testing

This question was designed to be answered narratively rather than as a result of a systematic review. It is devised to provide background information to the stakeholder.

Panel reactive antibody (PRA) testing seeks to evaluate who is most at risk of hyperacute or humoralrejection.[159] To orient the stakeholder, a PRA of eighty percent is supposed to reflect that the patient is crossmatch incompatible with 80 percent of donors. In general, patients with a PRA of more than 10 percent or more than 80 percent are considered sensitized or highly/broadly sensitized, respectively. However, different centers and investigators can use markedly different PRA cut offs for determining sensitized and highly/broadly sensitized. This system has been used since the 1960s in the United States.[159]

There are three types of assays used to determine PRA. The oldest is the Complement Dependent Cytotoxicity (CDC) test.[159,160] In this test, patient serum is tested against donor lymphocytes (B and T cells). Patients antibodies will coat antigen expressing lymphocytes and upon administration of complement to the serum, lymphocytes are killed and detected by cell stain. This method has several limitations. It only detects complement fixing antibodies (HLA Class I), detects non-HLA antigens, depends on lymphocyte and complement quality (acquisition and storage variability), and is limited by the cell panel used. As such, the CDC cannot be the only test of sensitization. The next type of assay is the Enzyme-Linked Immunoabsorbant Assay (ELISA) which is a solid phase assay which is more sensitive than the CDC. Available kits include the Quickscreen and QuickID which only detects HLA Class I antibodies and the B-Screen, LATM, and PRA-STAT which detects HLA Class I and II antibodies. The final type of assay is the flow cytometry test. There is the house method where locally acquired whole lymphocytes are used and a microbead method which uses purified HLA antigen coated microbeads. These methods allow determination of HLA Class I and II antibodies and specifies which HLA mismatches occur. Commerical kits include the Flow PRA and Luminextests. The CDC is thought to be inferior to the HLA Class I and II ELISA and microbead flow cytometry tests which are similar to each other.[159-161]

In two main evaluations, the ELISA and flow cytometry assays were found to be well correlated.[161,162] In the first study, two ELISA assay kits (Quickscreen (QS) and LATM (LATM)) were compared against each other and against a flow cytometrymicrobead kit (FlowPRA). The correlation in detecting HLA Class I and II antibodies were determined separately. The correlations between the findings between the different assay kits are given below:

ELISA Class I Assay (QS) with Flow Cytometry Class I (FPRAI); r = 0.72

ELISA Class I Assay (QS) with ELISA Class I Assay (LATMI); r = 0.81
Flow Cytometry Class I (FPRAI) with ELISA Class I (LATMI); r = 0.72
ELISA Class II Assay (QSB) with Flow Cytometry Class II (FPRAII); r = 0.87
ELISA Class II Assay (QSB) with ELISA Class I Assay (LATMII); r = 0.84
Flow Cytometry Class II (FPRAII) with ELISA Class I (LATMII); r = 0.89

So there was a strong correlation between two ELISA assay kits and with either ELISA kit versus the flow cytometry kit.[161] In the second study, an ELISA kit (PRA-STAT) was compared with a flow cytometry kit (Flowscreen) and with a CDC technique. The ELISA and flow cytometry assays for HLA Class I and II were well correlated (r=0.86, p<0.001). When evaluated in patients with graft failure, the correlation between these two assay types for HLA Class I and II was not as robust but still significant (r=0.49, p<0.001).In this population with graft failure, the correlation between CDC assay and the ELISA (r=0.28, p<0.001) or flow cytometry assay (r=0.30, p<0.001) for HLA Class I antibodies was low but still significant.CDC does not allow the determination of HLA Class II.[162] The CDC correlation to ELISA for Class I antibodies in this study is similar to that seen in two previous studies but not seen in a third.[163-165]

There are some fundamental problems with PRA testing. There are different types of assays and differences within assay classes which alter sensitivity and specificity. Forty-four percent of centers used peak PRA while 56 percent of centers use current PRA. The superiority of one approach over another is debatable but important since PRA may be altered in response to stimuli but may moderate over time.PRA response may be altered by the use of medications (rituximab, immune globulin, statins, cyclophosphamide/predisolone with plasmapheresis) or certain Angiotensin Converting Enzyme genotypes.[166-171] The composition of antigen panels can vary depending on the kit utilized or the cells that were locally procured. The antigen panels may differ in substantive ways from the donor population. Finally, even without altering PRA levels, the use of induction therapy with antithymocyte globulin might ameliorate or attenuate the negative impact of higher PRA levels on graft outcomes.

In one study, 241 transplanted patients were divided in to groups based on peak PRA levels.[172]Those with a peak PRA of 0-29 percent had better survival at one (90 percent vs. 79 percent, p<0.05) and three years (82 percent vs. 64 percent, p<0.05) than those with PRAs of 30-60percent.Detailed analysis of those in the higher peak PRA group found that better compatibility on the DR locus, a primary kidney transplant, a dialysis duration of less than 6 months, and the prophylactic use of antithymocyte globulin significantly improved graft outcome. This shows that the impact of PRA on outcomes is multifactorial in nature.

Calculated PRA Testing

In October 1, 2009, the United Network for Organ Sharing (UNOS) recommended against the current PRA system and for a calculated PRA (CPRA) system.[159] CPRA is based on the unacceptable HLA antigens to which patients are sensitized and which, if present in the donor, would represent an unacceptable risk for the candidate. CPRA has much greater applicability than traditional PRA because CPRA is based on HLA antigen frequencies among 12,000 kidney donors in the United States between 2003 and 2005 and represents the percentage of actual organ donors that express one or more unacceptable HLA antigens. If an HLA antibody is identified in a patient, a kidney with that antigen would not be offered. The higher the CPRA, the fewer kidneys would be offered. By March of 2009, only 13 of 256 kidney transplant centers did not enter specific HLA antigen incompatibilities into the UNOS system showing wide adoption.[159]

Impact of Sensitization on Eligibility for Transplantation

Of the 146 unique studies, 120 studies (82 percent) either did not report any sensitization results or evaluated sensitization results retrospectively only in those who received transplantation. As such, these data cannot be used to determine the impact of sensitization from transfusions on the ability to receive transplantation. The listing of these study results is included in Appendix E.

Twenty-six studies (18 percent) reported 37 analyses on the impact of transfusion on sensitization and its subsequent effect on eligibility for transplantation (Table 43). The sensitization rate in the 26 studies ranged from 1.9 percent to 45.5 percent, and it was assessed either based on the presence of cytotoxic antibodies or positive T-cell and/or B-cell crossmatches. Among sensitized patients, the percentage who were not subsequently transplanted with their planned kidney ranged from 0 percent to 100 percent. In many cases the outcomes of patients not originally transplanted were not given. However, where specified (Table 43), provides the known outcomes of these patients. In many cases, patients were subsequently transplanted although the time to transplant was prolonged, the type of kidney (cadaver versus living) given was different than originally planned, or patients were given interim therapy (plasmapheresis); although some patients died waiting for transplantation.

Of the 37 analyses: 10 analyses (27 percent) showed more sensitized patients were transplanted with their planned kidney than were not transplanted (including 6 analyses where all sensitized patients received transplantation)[19,52,77,95,102,131,135,173,174] while 21 analyses (57 percent),[14,30,65,70,86,92-94,97,99,103,104,108,122,132,133,136] found that more patients were precluded from receiving their planned transplantations (including 19 analyses where all sensitized patients were not transplanted with their planned kidneys). The remaining six analyses were part of DST versus random transfusion studies and in the random transfusion arms, they did not report transplantation status in sensitized patients.[19,65,86,97,133,135]

Amongst the 37 analyses, 21 and 16 analyses reported sensitization outcomes on subgroups of patients who received DST and other non-DST transfusions, respectively. Eighteen of the 21 DST (86 percent) analyses[14,19,30,65,70,86,92-94,97,99,104,108,122,132,133,136] found that more sensitized patients were precluded from transplantation with their planned kidneys, while this was seen only in 3 of the 16 (19 percent) non-DST analyses.[103,122,132]

Table 43. The impact of sensitization on the eligibility for transplantation in transfused patients

Study, Year (N=)	Type of transfusion	Number of transfused patients ($N_T=$)	Assessment	Number of transfused patients who were sensitized N_S/N_T (%)	Number of sensitized patients who were transplanted with planned kidney n/Ns (%)	Number of sensitized patients who were not transplanted with planned kidney n/Ns (%)	Comments
Jovicic S, 2010 (N=272)	DST RT	22 132	DST: presence of donor-specific antibodies RT: NR	3/22 (13.6) NR	0/3 (0) NR	3/3 (100) NR	*DST*: Of the 3 patients not transplanted with the planned grafts, 1 received cadaveric transplant, and 2 remained on HD *RT*: NR
Aalten J, 2009 (N=859)	DST mPTF RT	100 86 620	Presence of anti-HLA antibodies in the CDC	27/100 (27.0) 7/86 (8.1) 131/620 (21.1)	2/27 (7.4) 6/7 (85.7) NR	25/27 (92.6) 1/7 (14.3) NR	*DST & mPTF*: Kidney transplantations from the intended living donor were cancelled
Marti HP, 2006 (N=110)	DST	61	Sensitization: positive T-cell crossmatch	6/61 (9.8)	0/6 (0)	6/6 (100)	Of the 6 patients not transplanted with the planned grafts, 5 received cadaveric transplants instead of living transplants without delay, and 1 was lost to follow-up
Sakagami K, 1992 (N=109)	DST	57	T-cell crossmatch	4/57 (7.0)	0/4 (0)	4/4 (100)	Of the 4 patients not transplanted with the planned grafts, all were placed on cadaveric waiting list
Potter DE, 1991 (N=739)	DST RT	105 453	T-cell crossmatch	22/105 (21.0)* NR	0/22 (0) NR	22/22 (100) NR	*DST*: NR *RT*: NR
Reed A, 1991 (N=127)	DST RT	74 53	Crossmatch	7/74 (9.5) 1/53 (1.9)	0/7 (0) 0/1 (0)	7/7 (100) 1/1 (100)	*DST*: Of the 7 patients not transplanted with the planned grafts, 5 received cadaver transplant, 1 received HLA-identical living-related transplant, 1 did not receive any transplant *RT*: 1 received cadaver transplant
Salvatierra O, 1991 (N=118)	DST	71	NR	6/71 (8.4)	6/6 (100)	0/6 (0)	NA

Study, Year (N=)	Type of transfusion	Number of transfused patients ($N_T=$)	Assessment	Number of transfused patients who were sensitized Ns/N_T (%)	Number of sensitized patients who were transplanted with planned kidney n/Ns (%)	Number of sensitized patients who were not transplanted with planned kidney n/Ns (%)	Comments
Sells RA, 1989 (N=171)	DST RT	81 37	A permanent antidonor T cell or B cell antibody	12/81 (14.8) NR	0/12 (0) NR	12/12 (100) NR	Outcomes not reported for the 12 patients who were not transplanted
Casadei DH, 1987 (N=46)	DST	26	Crossmatch	2/26 (7.7)	0/2 (0)	2/2 (100)	Outcomes not reported for the 2 patients who were not transplanted
Cheigh JS, 1987 (N=60)	DST	60	Donor-specific lymphocytotoxic antibodies	5/60 (8.3)	0/5 (0)	5/5 (100)	Outcomes not reported for the 5 patients who were not transplanted
Huprikar AG, 1987 (N=66)	DST RT	33 33	Cytotoxic lymphocyte crossmatch	3/33 (9.1) 4/33 (12.1)	0/3 (0) 0/4 (0)	3/3 (100) 4/4 (100)	*DST*: Of the 3 patients not transplanted with the planned grafts, 2 delayed transplant by 1-2 weeks, and 1 had plasmapheresis, then transplant *RT*: All 4 patients delayed transplants by 2-8 weeks
Salvatierra O, 1987 a[†] (N=493)	DST	184	A positive T warm crossmatch or a positive B warm crossmatch with a concomitant positive fluorescence-activated cell sorter crossmatch	44/184 (23.9)	0/44 (0)	44/44 (100)	Outcomes not reported for the 44 patients who were not transplanted
Takahashi K, 1987 (N=290)	DST RT	171 119	T cells and (warm and cold) B cells crossmatch	21/171 (12.3)[‡] NR	21/21 (100) NR	0/21 (0) NR	*DST*: NA *RT*: NA
Leivestad T, 1986 (N=151)	DST	52	Persistent cytotoxic antibodies to donor T and B cells	9/52 (17.3)	0/9 (0)	9/9 (100)	Of the 9 patients not transplanted with the planned grafts, 1 received alternative live donor transplant, and 8 received cadaver transplant after waiting 2-42 months

Study, Year (N=)	Type of transfusion	Number of transfused patients (N$_T$=)	Assessment	Number of transfused patients who were sensitized Ns/N$_T$ (%)	Number of sensitized patients who were transplanted with planned kidney n/Ns (%)	Number of sensitized patients who were not transplanted with planned kidney n/Ns (%)	Comments
Glass NR, 1985 (N=250)	DST DST+AZA RT	62 113 75	Donor leukocyte crossmatch	19/62 (30.6) 16/113 (14.2) NR	0/19 (0) 0/16 (0) NR	19/19 (100) 16/16 (100) NR	Outcomes reported include patients who were sensitized and those with "unsuitable donors."
Sommer BG, 1985 (N=49)	DST	32	Cross-match testing against donor T- and B-lymphocytes Transplant done only with negative crossmatch	3/32 (9.4)	0/3 (0)	3/3 (100)	2 of the 3 patients received cadaver transplants, and the remaining patient had DST stopped & received original donor transplant
Akiyama N, 1984 (N=81)	DST	63	Cross-match	8/63 (12.7)	6/8 (75.0)	2/8 (25.0)	Of the 2 patients not transplanted with the planned grafts, 1 not transplanted due to positive crossmatch, and the other patient received graft after some period of time
Gardner B, 1984 (N=100)	RT	75	NR	16/75 (21.3)	16/16 (100)	0/16 (0)	NA
Sijpkens YWJ, 1984 (N=59)	DST	33	Crossmatch; PRA	15/33 (45.5)‡	0/15 (0)	15/15 (100)	Of the 15 patients not transplanted with the planned grafts, 4 received permanent dialysis, another 4 received cadaver transplant, and 7 patients awaited cadaver transplant
Nubé MJ, 1983 (N=55)	PT RT	15 26	Antibody positive : >5% reactive with panel	4/15 (26.7) 11/26 (42.3)	4/4 (100) 11/11 (100)	0/4 (0) 0/11 (0)	NA NA
d'Apice AJ, 1982 (N=63)	RT	63	Development of lymphocytotoxic antbodies to 10% or more of the panel	20/63 (31.7)	18/20 (90.0)	2/20 (10.0)	Of the 2 patients not transplanted with the planned grafts, 1 was refused for transplant, and the other patient remained on dialysis

Study, Year (N=)	Type of transfusion	Number of transfused patients (N_T=)	Assessment	Number of transfused patients who were sensitized Ns/N_T (%)	Number of sensitized patients who were transplanted with planned kidney n/Ns (%)	Number of sensitized patients who were not transplanted with planned kidney n/Ns (%)	Comments
Takahashi I, 1982 (N=40)	DST	24	Antibodies for donor T and B lymphocytes	1/24 (4.2)	0/1 (0)	1/1 (100)	Outcomes not reported for the patient who was not transplanted
Salvatierra O, 1980 (N=45)	DST	45	Crossmatch (cold and warm T- and B-lymphocytes)	13/45 (28.9)‡	0/13 (0)	13/13 (100)	Of the 13 patients not transplanted with the planned grafts, 4 patients received cadaver transplant. Outcomes not reported for remaining 9 patients
Solheim BG, 1980 (N=395)	RT	196	Lymphocytotoxic antibodies	48/196 (24.5)	32/48 (66.7)	16/48 (33.3)	Of the 16 patients not transplanted with the planned grafts, 14 died, and 2 were on a waiting list
Solheim BG, 1980 (N=191)	RT	85	Crossmatch; Presence of HLA antibodies	11/85 (10.6) [described as having HLA antibodies]	0/11 (0)	7/11 (63.6)	Outcomes for 4 patients not reported (transplant status unknown) Of the 7 patients who not transplanted with the planned grafts, 3 received cadaver transplant, another 3 still waiting for cadaver transplant, and 1 patient died while waiting for cadaver transplant
Opelz G, 1973 (N=144)	RT	144	Cytotoxicity positive: ≥5% reactivity against random donor panel	63/144 (43.8)	63/63 (100)	0/63 (0)	NA

* Sensitization based on positive crossmatch
† Salvatierra 1987a included a subgroup of transfused population whose crossmatches were performed
‡ Patients with a positive Tcell crossmatch or persistant positive warm Bcell crossmatch were considered as sensitized.

Anti-PBL=antiperipheral blood lymphocytes, CD=cadaveric donor transplantation, CMTSG=Canadian Multicenter Transplant Group, DST=donor specific transfusion, HLA=human leukocyte antigen, LD=living donor transplantation, LP=leukocyte-poor transfusions, mPTF=matched pretransplant transfusion, PRC=packed red cell transfusion, PT=protocol transfusion, RT=random transfusion, NA=not applicable, N=Total number of study population, n=number of patients in the subgroup, NR=not reported, NT=Number of transfused patients, Ns=number of sensitized patients

Key Question 2b. How useful are PRA assays in predicting sensitization from blood transfusions, donor specific antigen (DSA) sensitization, and renal transplant rejection/survival—especially in the setting of Q2a?

Univariate Analysis Results

Rejection

Two studies with two analyses evaluated the impact of PRA on graft rejection (Table 44).[35,175] In both analyses, the risk of rejection was not significantly elevated for the higher PRA group but was qualitatively lower when lower PRA groups were compared with higher PRA groups. Thus, we concluded that lower PRA is associated with a non-significant effect on rejection and graded the strength of the body of evidence as low.

Graft Survival

Fourteen studies with eighteen analyses evaluated the impact of different PRA levels (Table 45). Eleven of these analyses evaluated graft survival at 1-year[24,24,41,45,109,149,173-177] and all 18 of these analyses evaluated maximum duration graft survival (Table 45). In many cases, the use of peak or current PRA was not specified.

The 1-year graft survival was significantly better with lower versus higher PRA levels in four of eight (50.0 percent)[109,175,177] analyses that assessed for significance and not significantly different in the other analyses. The 1-year graft survival, where the direction of effect regardless of significance was assessed, for the lower PRA groups had higher graft survival in 10 of 11 (90.9 percent) analyses and lower survival in 1 of 11 (9.1 percent)[41] analyses. We concluded that lower PRA is associated with a beneficial to neutral effect on 1-year graft survival and graded the strength of the body of evidence as low.

The maximum duration graft survival was significantly better with lower versus higher PRA levels in 5 of 14 (35.7 percent) analyses that assessed for significance and not significantly different in the other analyses. The maximum duration graft survival, where the direction of effect regardless of significance was assessed, for the lower PRA groups had higher graft survival in 16 of 18 (88.9 percent) analyses and lower survival in 2 of 18 (11.1 percent) analyses. We concluded that lower PRA is associated with a beneficial to neutral effect on maximum duration graft survival and graded the strength of the body of evidence as low.

Patient Survival

One study with two analyses evaluated the impact of different PRA levels (Table 46).[53] Neither of these analyses evaluated the patient survival at 1 year and both of these analyses evaluated maximum duration of patient survival. The maximum duration patient survival was not significantly better for the lower PRA groups. We concluded that lower PRA is associated with a neutral effect on maximum duration patient survival and graded the strength of the body of evidence as low.

Multivariate Analysis Results

Seven studies were conducted evaluating the multivariate predictors of rejection, graft survival, or patient survival (Table 47). One study with two analyses (one for current and one for peak PRA) evaluated for rejection[122] and neither found that having a PRA >40 percent was an independent predictor of rejection. Seven analyses from six studies evaluated for graft survival[84,87,123,124,128,153] and in four analyses (57.1 percent),[123,124,128,153] having a lower PRA was a multivariate predictor of better graft survival. In the other three analyses,[85,87] having a lower PRA was not an independent predictor of graft survival and in no cases was it an independent predictor or worse graft survival. Three analyses[124,128] evaluated for patient survival and in one of the three (33.3 percent),[124] having a lower PRA was an independent predictor of better patient survival. In the other two cases,[128] it was not an independent predictor of patient survival and in no case was it an independent predictor of worse patient survival.

Table 44. Evidence depicting the association between PRA assays in predicting rejection (KQ 2b)

Study, Year (n)	Study Design	Transfused	PRA cut-off (%)	Rejection (%) 12 Months	Rejection (%) Max	Results
De Mattos, 1999 (N=108)	RO	Heterogeneous	Peak PRA ≤ 2 Peak PRA >2	NR	44 52 Followup NR P = 0.6	The incidence of rejection episodes was not significantly increased in the Peak PRA >2 group in comparison to the Peak PRA ≤2 group
Albrechtsen, 1987 (N=214)	CCT	Heterogeneous	PRA <10 PRA >10	46 69 P = NS	46 69 Followup 1 Year P = NS	The incidence of rejection episodes was not significantly increased in the PRA >10 group in comparison to the PRA <10 group

CCT = controlled clinical trial; NR = not reported, NS = not significant; P=p-value; PRA = Panel Reactive Antibodies; RO = retrospective observational

Table 45. Evidence depicting the association between PRA assays in predicting graft survival (KQ 2b)

Study, Year (n)	Study Design	Transfused	PRA cut-off (%)	Graft Survival (%) 12 Months	Graft Survival (%) Max	Results
Opelz, 2005a * (N=4,048)	RO	Heterogeneous	Negative PRA 1-50 PRA >50	83 80 72 P < 0.0001	72 63 56 Followup 10 - Year P < 0.0001	Graft survival **significantly** better for PRA negative group at 1 year and 10 years
Opelz, 2005b † (N=160,486)	RO	Heterogeneous	Negative PRA 1-50 PRA >50	95 94 93 P = 0.0831	48 40 See footnote‡ Followup 10 - Year P = < 0.0001	Graft survival better for "PRA Negative" but not significant at 1 year Graft survival significantly better for PRA negative group at 10 year
Albrechtsen, 1987 (N=214)	CCT	Heterogeneous	PRA <10 PRA >10	93 69 P < 0.01	93 69 Followup 1-Year P < 0.01	Graft survival **significantly** better for PRA <10 group at 1 year

Study, Year (n)	Study Design	Transfused	PRA cut-off (%)	Graft Survival (%) 12 Months	Graft Survival (%) Max	Results
Bucin, 1988a (N=116)	RO	Yes	Antibodies absent§ Antibodies present§	NR	49 63 Followup 2-Year P=NR	Graft survival worse for "antibodies absent" but with no statistical analysis at 2 years
Bucin, 1988b (N=116)	RO	No	Antibodies absent § Antibodies present §	NR	61 50 Followup 2-Year P=NR	Graft survival better for "antibodies absent" group but with no statistical analysis at 2 years
Alarif, 1987 (N=121)	RO	Yes	PRA <10 PRA ≥10	NR	90 63 Followup NR P = 0.011	Graft survival **significantly** better for PRA <10 group at not specified time point
Betuel, 1982 (N=278)	RO	Heterogeneous	Negative PRA 5-50 PRA >50	81 78 74 P = NR	74 66 NR Followup 2 Year P=NS	Graft survival better for "PRA Negative" but with no statistical analysis at 1 year Graft survival better for "PRA Negative" but not significant at 2 years
d'Apice, 1982 (N= 54)	RO	Yes	PRA <10 PRA ≥10	68 55 P = NS	65 55 Followup 1.5 Year P=NS	Graft survival better for PRA <10 but not significant at 1 and 1.5 year
Cho, 1983 (N= 647)	RO	Yes	PRA <10 PRA 10-50 PRA >50	74 67 48 P = NS	74 62 48 Followup 2 Year P=NS	Graft survival better for PRA <10 but not significant at 1 year and 2 year
De Mattos, 1999 (N= 108)	RO	Heterogeneous	Peak PRA ≤ 2 Peak PRA >2	NR	76 75 Followup 10 Year P = 0.9	Graft survival better for PRA ≤2 but not significant at 10 years

Study, Year (n)	Study Design	Transfused	PRA cut-off (%)	Graft Survival (%) 12 Months	Graft Survival (%) Max	Results
Feduska, 1981 (N= 732)	RO	Heterogeneous	PRA 0-10 PRA 11-50 PRA >50	50 52 61 P=NR	34 24 36 Followup 5 Year P=NR	Graft survival better for >50 than lower levels with no statistical analysis at 1 year and 5 years
Flechner, 1982 (N= 100)	RO	Heterogeneous	PRA < 10 PRA > 10	67 56 P=NS	67 56 Followup 1 Year P=NS	Graft survival better for PRA <10 but not significant at 1 year
Garvin, 1983a (N= 118)	RO	Heterogeneous	PRA < 10 PRA > 10	NR	58.3 50 Followup NR P=NS	Graft survival better for PRA <10 but not significant
Garvin, 1983b (N= 118)	RO	Heterogeneous	PRA < 10 PRA > 10	NR	73.3 50 Followup NR P=NS	Graft survival better for PRA <10 but not significant
Opelz, 1973 (N= 144)	RO	Yes	PRA <5 PRA ≥ 5	NR	47 6 Followup NR P<0.001	Graft survival significantly better for PRA <5 at non specified time point
Opelz, 1972 (N= 829)	RO	NR	PRA <5 PRA ≥ 5	55 36 P = NR	52 30 Followup 1.5 Year P = NR	Graft survival better for PRA <5 but with no statistical analysis at 1 and 1.5 year
Takiff, 1988a (N= 33,594)	RO	Heterogeneous	Curent PRA 0-10 Curent PRA 11-20 Curent PRA 21-50 Curent PRA >50	61 62 62 57 P < 0.025	30 30 31 23 Followup 10 Year P=NS	Graft survival **significantly** better for Current PRA <50 groups at 1 year but not at 10 year

Study, Year (n)	Study Design	Transfused	PRA cut-off (%)	Graft Survival (%) 12 Months	Graft Survival (%) Max	Results
Takiff, 1988b (N= 33,594)	RO	Heterogeneous	Peak PRA 0-10	62	27	Graft survival **significantly** better for Peak PRA <50 groups at 1 year but not at 10 year
			Peak PRA 11-20	60	30	
			Peak PRA 21-50	61	28	
			Peak PRA >50	55	22	
				P <0.005	Followup 10 Year P=NS	

* Cadaver kidney transplant populations
† HLA-identical sibling transplant populations
‡ Cannot be extrapolated from the figure
§ Study reported results of presence or absence of antibody assessed by local panel of donors

CCT = controlled clinical trial; N = number; NR = not reported; NS = not significant; P=p value; PRA = Panel Reactive Antibodies; RO = retrospective observational

Table 46. Evidence depicting the association between PRA assays in predicting patient survival (KQ 2b)

Study, Year (n)	Study Design	Transfused	PRA cut-off (%)	Patient Survival (%) 12 Months	Patient Survival (%) Max	Results
Garvin, 1983a (N= 118)	RO	Heterogeneous	PRA < 10 PRA > 10	NR	92.3 91.6 Followup NR P=NS	Patient survival better for PRA <10 but not significant
Garvin, 1983b (N= 118)	RO	Heterogeneous	PRA < 10 PRA > 10	NR	93.7 92.3 Followup NR P=NS	Patient survival better for PRA <10 but not significant

n=number; NR = not reported; NS = not significant; P=p value; PRA = Panel Reactive Antibodies; RO = retrospective observational

Table 47. Multivariate results depicting the association between PRA assays in predicting renal transplant outcomes (KQ 2b)

Study, Year (n)	Study Design	Analysis Type	Other Variables	PRA cut-off	Evaluated Outcomes	Multivariate Results (95% CI)	Multivariate P-value
Tang, 2008 (N= 2882)	RO	Cox proportional hazard model	Extensive number	Peak PRA level (each 10% increase)	Graft Failure	HR 1.06 (1.03-1.10)	P < 0.001
					Recipient Death	HR 1.04 (1.00-1.07)	P < 0.05
Opelz, 2005 (N= 164,534)	RO	Cox's regression analysis	Transplant Number Year of transplantation Immunosuppression Donor & recipient age, sex and race Pre-tx transfusion	PRA 1-50% vs. PRA negative before transplantation	Graft Loss	RR 1.29 (1.09-1.53)	P = 0.003
				PRA > 50 vs. PRA negative before transplantation	Graft Loss	RR 1.87 (1.47-2.37)	P < 0.0001

Study, Year (n)	Study Design	Analysis Type	Other Variables	PRA cut-off	Evaluated Outcomes	Multivariate Results (95% CI)	Multivariate P-value
Bunnapradist, 2003 (N= 7079)	RO	Cox regression analysis	Recipient age >55 Male Pre-Tx transfusion Donor age HLA mismatch	PRA > 30%	Graft Failure	HR 1.39 (1.06-1.81)	0.016
Poli, 1995 (N= 416)	RO	Cox model stepwise regression	HLA-DRB1 HLA-A,B Donor age Graft number Pre-tx transfusioin	PRA 0 (0, >0)	Graft Survival	RR 1.3 (0.6-2.8)	0.6
Reed, 1991 (N= 127)	RO	Cox proportional hazards; Poisson random variable methods	DST Pregnancy Age Sex AB match DR match Prior transplant	Baseline PRA > 40% Peak PRA > 40%	Rejection Rejection	NR NR	P = 0.73 P = 0.91
Sanfilippo, 1986 (N= 3811)	RO	Cox regression model	Extensive number	Peak PRA ≥ 60%	Graft failure	RR 1.346 (NR)	0.003
CMTSG, 1986 (N= 291)	CCT	Cox proportional-hazards model	Extensive number	Current PRA >10%	Patient Death	RR 1.28 (NR)	NS
					Graft Loss	RR 2.29 (NR)	P < 0.05
				Highest PRA >50%	Patient Death	RR 1.15 (NR)	NS
					Graft Loss	RR 1.45 (NR)	NS
Rao, 1983 (N= 300)	RO	Exploratory multivariate regression analysis	Extensive number	PRA ≥ 50%	Graft Survival	RR NR (NR) (unfavorable effect)	P = 0.10

CCT= controlled clinical trial; CMTSG=Canadian Multicenter Transplant Study Group, DST= donor specific transfusion; HLA-A,B= human leukocyte antigen-AB; HLA-DRB= human leukocyte antigen DRB; HR= hazard ratio; N= number; NR=not reported; NS= not significant; P= p-value; PRA= Panel Reactive Antibodies; RO= retrospective observational; RR= relative risk; Tx= transfusion

Discussion

Although we evaluated a voluminous literature set, the studies were predominantly retrospective, did not account for confounding, and in many cases had sparse reporting of demographics. The studies also had very high clinical and methodological heterogeneity precluding the ability to pool results. This heterogeneity was due to the different definitions of endpoints of interest, differing subpopulations of patients, different etiologies of renal failure, studies with and without any HLA-matching, differing cold ischemia times, the use of or different mixture of living versus deceased donors, use of perioperative transfusion, previous transplant or pregnancy history, history of previous random transfusions in patients receiving DST, differing followup periods, and ABO blood incompatibilities. This high degree of clinical and methodological heterogeneity precluded the ability to pool the results.

We chose to evaluate our data based on the percentage of analyses evaluating an endpoint that either showed a significant effect (either beneficial or detrimental) or a non-significant effect. We then evaluated our data based on the direction and/or magnitude of effect (either beneficial or detrimental). This approach has limitations because analyses of varying quality and sample size were evaluated together but it provides that only type of independent qualitative analyses that can be done on such a literature base.

In the vast majority of analyses reporting the significance of their findings, the use of transfusions versus no transfusions either resulted in a significantly beneficial or insignificant effect on rejection, graft survival, or patient survival. When analyses were evaluated regardless of the significance of the findings, which allows underpowered analyses and analyses for which the original study authors did not discern the significance of their findings to be included, we found that the use of transfusions versus no transfusions either resulted in either beneficial or small/null effects on rejection, graft survival, or patient survival. For the analyses evaluating the impact of the use of larger number of transfusion/transfused units versus no, or a smaller number of transfused/transfused units, we found mixed effects on rejection, graft survival, or patient survival. So the literature, weak as it is, demonstrates a neutral to positive effect resulting from transfusion and does not reflect a detrimental effect resulting from transfusion. The same results were found when comparing DST with non-DST transfusions or leukocyte depleted/free transfusions with no or non-leukocyte depleted/free transfusions with either neutral or beneficial effects resulting.

In our technology assessment, having a lower PRA due to transfusion generally has a beneficial to neutral effect on outcomes. These data are limited because it does not consistently define PRA in the same manner (Peak or Current PRA), does not allow assessment for the specific HLA antibodies that the patients are incompatible with (like is becoming the standard of care with "calculated PRA"), the assays for PRA have inter and intra-assay variability, there are modulators of PRA level and the use of these modulators are not specified in the studies, the time course from exposure to transfusion or other stimuli to the time the PRA is recorded is not defined, and most importantly that the degree to which the elevated PRA in these studies were due to transfusions versus other stimuli such as transplants or other factors such as pregnancy cannot be determined. It should be noted that PRA is a surrogate measure for immunization, and its link to renal allograft outcomes is tenuous due to the myriad confounding factors such as donor types, immunosuppression used, and other factors that can influence the transplant outcomes. The purpose of this TA is not to identify a specific causal link between PRA and renal allograft outcomes, but rather to examine the available data to identify the correlation between the two in studies that did assess transfusion use and final health outcomes.

There are problems with internal validity and heterogeneity with these individual studies. As such, we have low confidence that the evidence reflects the true effect. Further research is likely to change our confidence in the estimate of effect and likely change the estimate as well. In addition, the findings of our technology assessment need to be viewed in light of one very important limitation. The studies, as devised, evaluated the impact of transfusions on transplantation outcomes but could only be determined among those patients who actually received transplantation. In several of our included studies, we found that a proportion of patients who were sensitized after transfusion ended up not being considered for their planned kidney and had a delay in transplantation, received a different organ type (deceased versus living), had to undergo a procedure to attenuate sensitization such as plasmapheresis, or went back on the waiting list. In some cases, patients reportedly died while on the waiting list. As such, we cannot be sure that transfusions have a beneficial to neutral effect on transplantation outcomes or select out those most likely to be successful after transplantation. It is unclear why intention-to-treat analyses were not utilized by investigators, where possible.

There are data from large registries that are published in non-peer reviewed book chapters, do not have an adequate description of methods, and in most cases do not account for a myriad of confounders. While they did not make our *a priori* criteria for study inclusion, they do provide provocative data that should be noted. There are at least six book chapters within the Clinical Transplants textbook that uses data from the UCLA or UNOS registries. In one book chapter using the UCLA Transplant Registry over a ten year period (1981 to 1990), the 1-year graft survival in patients undergoing first transplants was significantly better in unsensitized patients (PRA 0-10%) versus those with a PRA >50% in 5 of the 10 years.[7] In the same book chapter, using data from the UCLA Transplant Registry from 1985 to 1990 or the UNOS Registry from 1987 to 1990 (the source of the evidence was not specified), the authors found that receiving more transfusions increased the number of patients undergoing a first transplant becoming sensitized. Given these two pieces of indirect evidence, it would seem intuitive that transfusions would negatively impact 1-year graft survival but like the analyses that made it into our Technology Assessment, transfusions either had a beneficial or neutral effect in both males and females who had a PRA of 0-10%, PRA of 11-50%, or PRA of >50%. Clearly there is a disconnect in logic that may suggest: (1) the benefits of reducing graft rejection through a non-PRA mechanism of transfusion overcomes the negative effect of raising PRA on graft rejection; (2) transfusions self-select those with the greater ability to do well after transplantation; or (3) another confounder explains the discrepancy but has not been evaluated. It is possible that the avoidance of incompatible organs attenuates the negative impact of elevated PRA on outcomes but in so doing, decreases the available pool of organs. This is plausible since in this book chapter, the waiting time for an organ is prolonged in both males and females when PRAs are elevated. Another chapter from this textbook using UNOS data from 1995 to 2000 shows that increasing the number of transfusions qualitatively increased the number of sensitized patients and reduced graft survival, although statistical analyses were not provided.[8] In book chapter from an earlier edition of the textbook, UNOS Registry data from 1988 to 1996 was reported. It reported that increasing numbers of transfusions significantly increased sensitization (higher PRAs) and that elevated PRA (from any cause) was qualitatively associated with worse graft survival although statistical results for this latter analysis were not provided.[9] In another book chapter, UCLA Registry data from 1981 to 1990 found qualitatively better 1-year graft survival annually from 1981 through 1987, similar 1-year graft survival from 1988 to 1989, and worse survival in 1990 in those with 1 or more transfusions versus no transfusions although the authors suggested that the 1990 data could be a spurious result produced by late reporting of followup.[10,178] UNOS Registry data from 1987 to 1990 found similar 1-year graft survival in those with 1 or more transfusions versus no transfusions. Another book chapter using UNOS data reiterated similar risks of higher numbers of transfusions increasing risk of developing higher PRAs and higher PRAs (from any source) increasing risk of graft failure[11] while another book chapter reiterated that patients with PRAs >50% (from any cause) have longer waiting times for transplantation.[12]

In the USRDS Annual Data Report in 2010, patients with higher PRAs have longer waiting times.[13] Receiving a transfusion while on the transplant waiting list is associated with a 5-fold higher risk of dying while on the wait list within the first five years and an 11% reduction in the likelihood of receiving a transplant within the first 5 years. Why such a disparity exists between the relatively small reduction in transplantation and the large increase in the likelihood of death of the waiting list is unclear. The data was adjusted for age, gender, race, ethnicity, cause of end stage renal disease, blood type, body mass index, pretransplant time on dialysis, education, dialysis type, and comorbid conditions. It could be that while the risk of having no transplant within 5 years is low, the prolongation of waiting time leads to poorer outcomes, there is ultimately a poorer match, or transfusion may be a marker of some other underlying disorder that hastens death unrelated to the transfused product itself. Ultimately, these data that were not included in our results section supports our general findings about the implications of receiving transfusions in those who actually receive transplants and underscores the potential for adverse outcomes in those who are not ultimately transplanted due to sensitization.

While the data provided by USRDS on overall transplant outcomes is extensive, the USRDS report was not focused on the direct impact of transfusions on transplant outcomes. The USRDS data collection system is limited to self-reporting of transfusion status in transplant candidates and recipients, in which it is limited to discrete data (i.e. yes, no, or unknown) on whether patients have received transfusions while the indications and/or appropriateness of the transfusions are often unknown. As such, the direct correlation of sensitization and transfusion cannot be established.

Future Research Directions

We believe that additional adequately powered studies should be conducted. In these studies we believe that they should be multi-institutional because individual center practices and procedures are so variable, have adequate reporting of demographics and either use statistical means to account for confounders (propensity score adjustment or matching) or use of randomization, have standard definitions of outcomes, and have a standard followup time of at least 1-year. Patients receiving or being randomized to no transfusions should be screened to assure that this not only includes transfusions within the dialysis or transplant center but other transfusions as well. We believe that standard PRA testing should be supplanted with updated CPRA testing so that specific HLA antigen sensitivities resulting from transfusions can be identified and perhaps correlated with outcomes. Outcomes such as sensitization rate, access to transplantation, and waiting time to transplantation during the pretransplant time period as well as graft outcomes during post-transplant period should be evaluated.

The impact of different immunosuppressive regimens (induction and maintenance as well as novel therapies such as statins) on outcomes in patients receiving transfusions to identify those regimens which can suppress the advantageous or detrimental effects of transfusion on outcomes is needed. This should be specifically evaluated to determine whether transfusions need to be encouraged, avoided, or matched with certain regimens. Such evaluations should adhere to good study conduction practices.

Data from large scale registries could be used for future research but should be published in peer reviewed journals, have an adequate use and description of methods, have a reliable and objective data collection system, as well as account for a myriad of confounders.

Conclusion

The conclusions to the key questions of this technology assessment and the grading of the strength of the body of evidence are summarized in Table 48.

Unlike prior renal transplants which seem to worsen renal allograft outcomes, transfusions generally have beneficial to neutral effects on renal allograft outcomes, and have minimal detrimental effects on the outcomes for renal transplant recipients. There is not much support for the notion that transfusions increase the risk of graft rejection among those receiving transplantation. Although there is evidence that patients receiving pretransplant transfusions have increased levels of sensitization as assessed by PRA, the relationship between the number of pretransplant transfusions and the extent of levels of sensitization is still not established. It should be noted that in some studies, patients who were candidates for transplantation were ultimately not offered the transplant due to high PRA levels. Some other studies did not disclose the number of patients who were ultimately not transplanted due to a high PRA as they focused on the population undergoing transplant. This is a major confounder in these studies.

When we examine results based on advancing time periods (before 1942, 1984–1991, and 1992 to the present), the percentage of analyses showing benefit is attenuated in more recently conducted studies. With regard to rejection, the data are more ambiguous with some analyses showing benefit, some showing a neutral effect, and other analyses showing harm, although the number of studies evaluating more recent time periods is quite limited.

In essence, the literature base is weak and future research conducted with proper control for confounders, disclosure of baseline characteristics, and use of other good study design techniques is needed to assess the impact of transfusions on allograft and patient survival outcomes in renal transplant recipients.

Table 48. Overview of Study Outcomes

Outcome	Total Number of Analyses	Conclusion	Strength of Evidence
KEY QUESTION 1a ENDPOINTS			
REJECTION:		Transfusion has a:	
Significant Findings	25	Beneficial to no significant effect on rejection	Low
Direction of Effect	47	Beneficial to no effect on rejection	Insufficient
1-YR GRAFT SURVIVAL:		Transfusion has a:	
Significant Findings	55	Beneficial to no significant effect on graft survival	Low
Magnitude of Effect	132	Large beneficial impact or small impact on graft survival	Low
MAX DURATION GRAFT SURVIVAL:		Transfusion has a:	
Significant Findings	65	Beneficial to no significant effect on graft survival	Low
Magnitude of Effect	146	Large beneficial impact or small impact on graft survival	Low
1-YR PATIENT SURVIVAL:		Transfusion has a:	
Significant Findings	16	Beneficial to no significant effect on patient survival	Low
Magnitude of Effect	35	Large beneficial impact or small impact on patient survival	Low
MAX DURATION PATIENT SURVIVAL:		Transfusion has a:	
Significant Findings	18	Beneficial to no significant effect on patient survival	Low
Magnitude of Effect	41	Large beneficial impact or small impact on patient survival	Low
MULTIVARIATE ANALYSES:		The covariate has:	
Prior Transplant	22	Detrimental to no significant effect on rejection, graft survival, and patient survival	Low
Transfusion	13	Beneficial to no significant effect on rejection and graft survival	Low
Pregnancy	5	Beneficial effect on rejection but detrimental to no significant effect on graft survival	Insufficient (rejection), Low (Graft Survival)
KEY QUESTION 1b i ENDPOINTS			
REJECTION:		DST Transfusion has a:	
Significant Findings	3	Beneficial to no significant effect on rejection	Low
Direction of Effect	7	Beneficial to no effect on rejection	Insufficient
1-YR GRAFT SURVIVAL:		Transfusion has a:	
Significant Findings	4	Beneficial to no significant effect on graft survival	Low
Magnitude of Effect	16	Large beneficial impact or small impact on graft survival	Low

Outcome	Total Number of Analyses	Conclusion	Strength of Evidence
MAX DURATION GRAFT SURVIVAL:		Transfusion has a:	
Significant Findings	5	Beneficial to no significant effect on graft survival	Low
Magnitude of Effect	17	Large beneficial impact or small impact on graft survival	Low
1-YR PATIENT SURVIVAL:		Transfusion has a:	
Significant Findings	2	Non-significant effect on patient survival	Insufficient
Magnitude of Effect	4	Small impact on patient survival	Low
MAX DURATION PATIENT SURVIVAL:		Transfusion has a:	
Significant Findings	2	Non-significant effect on patient survival	Insufficient
Magnitude of Effect	4	Small impact on patient survival	Low
MULTIVARIATE ANALYSES:		The covariate has:	
DST vs Non-DST	5	Beneficial to no significant effect on rejection or graft survival	Low
KEY QUESTION 1b ii ENDPOINTS			
REJECTION: NUMBER OF TRANSFUSIONS:		Versus a lower number of transfusions, a higher number of transfusions is:	
Significant Findings	5	Beneficial to no significant effect on rejection	Low
Direction of Effect	18	Beneficial to no effect on rejection	Insufficient
NUMBER OF UNITS TRANSFUSED:		Versus no units of blood transfused, increasing number of units:	
Significant Findings	1	Non-significant effect on rejection	Insufficient
Direction of Effect	1	No effect on rejection	Insufficient

Outcome	Total Number of Analyses	Conclusion	Strength of Evidence
1-YR GRAFT SURVIVAL: NUMBER OF TRANSFUSIONS VERSUS NO TRANSFUSION:			
Significant Findings	12	1-5, 5-10, or >10 transfusions versus no transfusions has a: Beneficial to no significant effect on graft survival	Low
Magnitude of Effect	51	Large beneficial impact or small impact on graft survival	Low
HIGHER VERSUS LOWER NUMBER OF TRANSFUSIONS:			
Significant Findings	11	≥5 vs. 1-5, ≥10 vs. 1-5, ≥10 vs. ≥5 transfusions has a: Beneficial to no significant effect on graft survival	Low
Magnitude of Effect	43	Large beneficial impact or small impact on graft survival	Low
NUMBER OF UNITS TRANSFUSED VERSUS NO TRANSFUSION:			
Significant Findings	11	1-5, 5-10, or >10 transfusions versus no transfusions has a: Beneficial to no significant effect on graft survival	Low
Magnitude of Effect	21	Large beneficial impact or small impact on graft survival	Low
HIGHER VERSUS LOWER NUMBER OF UNITS TRANSFUSED:			
Significant Findings	6	≥5 vs. 1-5, ≥10 vs. 1-5, ≥10 vs. ≥5 transfusions has a: Beneficial to no significant effect on graft survival	Low
Magnitude of Effect	12	Large beneficial impact or small impact on graft survival	Low

Outcome	Total Number of Analyses	Conclusion	Strength of Evidence
MAX DURATION GRAFT SURVIVAL:			
NUMBER OF TRANSFUSIONS VERSUS NO TRANSFUSION:		1-5, 5-10, or >10 transfusions versus no transfusions has a:	
Significant Findings	9	Beneficial to no significant effect on graft survival	Low
Magnitude of Effect	53	Large beneficial impact or small impact on graft survival	Low
HIGHER VERSUS LOWER NUMBER OF TRANSFUSIONS:		≥5 vs. 1-5, ≥10 vs. 1-5, ≥10 vs. ≥5 transfusions has a:	
Significant Findings	10	Beneficial to no significant effect on graft survival	Low
Magnitude of Effect	47	Large beneficial impact or small impact on graft survival	Low
NUMBER OF UNITS TRANSFUSED VERSUS NO TRANSFUSION:		1-5, 5-10, or >10 transfusions versus no transfusions has a:	
Significant Findings	16	Beneficial to no significant effect on graft survival	Low
Magnitude of Effect	22	Large beneficial impact or small impact on graft survival	Low
HIGHER VERSUS LOWER NUMBER OF UNITS TRANSFUSED:		≥5 vs. 1-5, ≥10 vs. 1-5, ≥10 vs. ≥5 transfusions has a:	
Significant Findings	12	Beneficial to no significant effect on graft survival	Low
Magnitude of Effect	16	Large beneficial impact or small impact on graft survival	Low
1-YR PATIENT SURVIVAL:			
NUMBER OF TRANSFUSIONS VERSUS NO TRANSFUSION:		1-5, 5-10, or >10 transfusions versus no transfusions has a:	
Significant Findings	8	Non-significant effect on patient survival	Low
Magnitude of Effect	8	Large beneficial impact or small impact on patient survival	Low
HIGHER VERSUS LOWER NUMBER OF TRANSFUSIONS:		≥5 vs. 1-5, ≥10 vs. 1-5, ≥10 vs. ≥5 transfusions has a:	
Significant Findings	7	No significant effect on patient survival	Low
Magnitude of Effect	7	Small impact on patient survival	Low

Outcome	Total Number of Analyses	Conclusion	Strength of Evidence
MAX DURATION PATIENT SURVIVAL:			
NUMBER OF TRANSFUSIONS VERSUS NO TRANSFUSION:		1-5, 5-10, or >10 transfusions versus no transfusions has a:	
Significant Findings	8	Non-significant effect on patient survival	Low
Magnitude of Effect	7	Large beneficial impact or small impact on patient survival	Low
HIGHER VERSUS LOWER NUMBER OF TRANSFUSIONS:		≥5 vs. 1-5, ≥10 vs. 1-5, ≥10 vs. ≥5 transfusions has a:	
Significant Findings	7	No significant effect on patient survival	Low
Magnitude of Effect	5	Small impact on patient survival	Low
MULTIVARIATE ANALYSES:			
Transfusion of Varying Numbers vs. No Transfusion	16	Transfusion has a: Detrimental to no significant effect on rejection or graft survival	Low
>5 transfusions vs. 1-5 transfusions	4	Versus 1-5 transfusions, >5 transfusions has a: Detrimental to neutral effect on rejection and graft survival	Low
KEY QUESTION 1b iii ENDPOINTS			
1-YR GRAFT SURVIVAL:			
LEUKOCYTE DEPLETED VS. NO TRANSFUSION		Versus no transfusion, leukocyte depleted transfusion has a:	
Magnitude of Effect	2	Large beneficial impact on graft survival	Low
LEUKOCYTE DEPLETED VS. TRANSFUSION:		Versus transfusion, leukocyte depleted transfusion has a:	
Significant Findings	1	Non-significant effect on graft survival	Insufficient
Magnitude of Effect	2	Small change in graft survival	Low
MAX DURATION GRAFT SURVIVAL:			
LEUKOCYTE DEPLETED VS. NO TRANSFUSION		Versus no transfusion, leukocyte depleted transfusion has a:	
Magnitude of Effect	2	Large beneficial impact on graft survival	Low
LEUKOCYTE DEPLETED VS. TRANSFUSION:		Versus transfusion, leukocyte depleted transfusion has a:	
Significant Findings	1	Non-significant effect on graft survival	Insufficient
Magnitude of Effect	2	Large beneficial effect or small change in graft survival	Low

Outcome	Total Number of Analyses	Conclusion	Strength of Evidence
MAX DURATION PATIENT SURVIVAL: LEUKOCYTE DEPLETED VS. NO TRANSFUSION			
Magnitude of Effect	1	No effect on rejection	Insufficient
LEUKOCYTE DEPLETED VS. TRANSFUSION:			
Significant Findings	1	No significant effect on rejection	Insufficient
Magnitude of Effect	1	No effect on rejection	Insufficient
KEY QUESTION 1b iv-v ENDPOINTS			
REJECTION:		Over progressive time periods transfusion has a:	
Significant Findings	11	Up to the year 1992, transfusion had a significant beneficial to neutral effect but after 1992, it may not have this effect	Low
Direction of Effect	35	Up to the year 1992, transfusion had a beneficial to neutral effect but after 1992, it may not have this effect	Low
1-YR GRAFT SURVIVAL:		Over progressive time periods transfusion has a:	
Significant Findings	47	Transfusion had a significant beneficial to neutral effect	Low
Magnitude of Effect	108	Transfusion has a large beneficial impact or small impact on graft survival	Low
MAX DURATION GRAFT SURVIVAL:		Over progressive time periods transfusion has a:	
Significant Findings	57	Transfusion had a significant beneficial to neutral effect	Low
Magnitude of Effect	119	Transfusion has a large beneficial impact or small impact on graft survival	Low
1-YR PATIENT SURVIVAL:		Over progressive time periods transfusion has a:	
Significant Findings	17	Transfusion had a significant beneficial to neutral effect	Low
Magnitude of Effect	30	Transfusion has a large beneficial impact or small impact on patient survival	Low
MAX DURATION PATIENT SURVIVAL:		Over progressive time periods transfusion has a:	
SignificantFindings	18	Transfusion had a significant beneficial to neutral effect	Low
Magnitude of Effect	37	Transfusion has a large beneficial impact or small impact on patient survival	Low
KEY QUESTION 2b ENDPOINTS			
REJECTION:		Lower PRA% is associated with a:	
Significant Findings	2	Non-significant effect on rejection	Low
Direction of Effect	2	Directionally less rejection	Insufficient

Outcome	Total Number of Analyses	Conclusion	Strength of Evidence
1-YR GRAFT SURVIVAL:		Lower PRA% is associated with a:	
Significant Findings	8	Significant beneficial to neutral effect	Low
Direction of Effect	11	Large beneficial impact or small impact on graft survival	Low
MAX DURATION GRAFT SURVIVAL:		Lower PRA% is associated with a:	
Significant Findings	14	Significant beneficial to neutral effect on graft survival	Low
Direction of Effect	18	Large beneficial impact or small impact on graft survival	Low
MAX DURATION PATIENT SURVIVAL:		Lower PRA% is associated with a:	
Significant Findings	2	Non-significant effect on patient survival	Low
MULTIVARIATE ANALYSES:		Lower PRA is:	
Rejection	2	Not an independent predictor of lower rejection	Low
Graft Survival	7	Significant beneficial to neutral effect of graft survival	Low
Patient Survival	3	Significant beneficial to neutral effect on patient survival	Low

PRA = Panel Reactive Antibodies, YR = Year

References

1. S. Gabardi and A. J. Olyaei. Solid organ transplantation, chapter 55. In, Chisolm-Burns MA, Ed. Pharmacotherapy Principles and Practice, Second Edition. McGraw-Hill, NY, NY. 2010: pgs 939-64.

2. The Organ Procurement and Transplant Network (OPTN). Available at: http://optn.transplant.hrsa.gov/latestdata/viewdatareports.asp. Accessed: July 6, 2010.

3. Opelz G, Sengar DP, Mickey MR, et al. Effect of blood transfusions on subsequent kidney transplants. TRANSPLANT PROC 1973;5:253-9. PMID: 4572098

4. Halloran PF. Call for revolution: a new approach to describing allograft deterioration. Am J Transplant 2002;2:195-200.PMID: 12096779

5. Opelz G, Terasaki PI. Improvement of kidney-graft survival with increased numbers of blood transfusions. N Engl J Med 1978;299:799-803. PMID: 357971

6. Fuller TC, Delmonico FL, Cosimi B, et al. Impact of blood transfusion on renal transplantation. Ann Surg 1978;187:211-8. PMID: 343736

7. Zhou YC, Cecka JM. Sensitization in renal transplantation. Clin Transpl 1991;313-23. PMID: 1820127

8. Hardy S, Lee SH, Terasaki PI. Sensitization 2001. Clin Transpl 2001;271-8. PMID: 12211790

9. Katznelson S, Bhaduri S, Cecka JM. Clinical aspects of sensitization. Clin Transpl 1997;285-96. PMID: 9919412

10. Ahmed Z, Pi T. Effect of transfusions. Clin Transpl 1991;305-12. PMID: 1820125

11. Cecka JM. The UNOS Scientific Renal Transplant Registry--2000. Clin Transpl 2000;1-18. PMID: 11512303

12. Cecka JM, Cho L. Sensitization. Clin Transpl 1988;365-73. PMID: 3154486

13. Collins AJ, Foley RN, Herzog C, et al. US Renal Data System 2010 Annual Data Report. Am J Kidney Dis 2011;57 (1 Suppl 1):e311-24.

14. Marti HP, Henschkowski J, Laux G, et al. Effect of donor-specific transfusions on the outcome of renal allografts in the cyclosporine era. Transpl Int 2006;19:19-26. PMID : 16359373

15. Hiesse C, Busson M, Buisson C, et al. Multicenter trial of one HLA-DR-matched or mismatched blood transfusion prior to cadaveric renal transplantation. Kidney Int 2001;60:341-9. PMID: 11422770

16. Alexander JW, Light JA, Donaldson LA, et al. Evaluation of pre- and posttransplant donor-specific transfusion/cyclosporine A in non-HLA identical living donor kidney transplant recipients. Cooperative Clinical Trials in Transplantation Research Group. Transplantation 1999;68:1117-24. PMID: 10551639

17. Opelz G, Vanrenterghem Y, Kirste G, et al. Prospective evaluation of pretransplant blood transfusions in cadaver kidney recipients. Transplantation 1997;63:964-7. PMID: 9112348

18. Sharma RK, Rai PK, Kumar A, et al. Role of preoperative donor-specific transfusion and cyclosporine in haplo-identical living related renal transplant recipients. Nephron 1997;75:20-4. PMID: 9031265

19. Aalten J, Bemelman FJ, van den Berg-Loonen EM, et al. Pre-kidney-transplant blood transfusions do not improve transplantation outcome: a Dutch national study. Nephrol Dial Transplant 2009;24:2559-66. PMID: 19474284

20. Albrechtsen D, Flatmark A, Brynger H, et al. Impact of blood transfusions and HLA matching on national kidney transplant programs: the first Swedish-Norwegian Study of cyclosporine. Transplant Proc 1988;20:257-60. PMID : 3291252

21. Barbari A, Stephan A, Masri MA, et al. Donor specific transfusion in kidney transplantation: effect of different immunosuppressive protocols on graft

outcome. Transplant Proc 2001;33:2787-8. PMID: 11498161

22. Barber WH. Donor-specific transfusions in renal transplantation. Clin Transplant 1994;8:204-6. PMID: 8019037

23. Basri N, Nezamuddin N, Aman H, et al. Donor-specific transfusion in living-related renal transplants. Transplant Proc 1992;24:1746. PMID : 1412822

24. Betuel H, Touraine JL, Malik MC, et al. Kidney transplantation in patients submitted to deliberate transfusions, to random transfusions, and to thoracic duct drainage. Transplant Proc 1982;14:276-8. PMID: 7051466

25. Blamey RW, Knapp MS, Burden RP, et al. Blood transfusion and renal allograft survival. Br Med J 1978;1:138-40. PMID: 339996

26. Briggs JD, Canavan JS, Dick HM, et al. Influence of HLA matching and blood transfusion on renal allograft survival. Transplantation 1978;25:80-5. PMID: 341429

27. Brynger H, Frisk B, Ahlmen J, et al. Graft survival and blood transfusion. Proc Eur Dial Transplant Assoc 1977;14:290-5. PMID: 341128

28. Brynger H, Persson H, Flatmark A, et al. No effect of blood transfusions or HLA matching on renal graft success rate in recipients treated with cyclosporine-prednisolone or cyclosporine-azathioprine-prednisolone: the Scandinavian experience. Transplant Proc 1988;20:261-3. PMID: 3291253

29. Bucin D. Adverse effect of blood transfusion on the long-term outcome of kidney transplantation. Exp Clin Immunogenet 1988;5:39-47. PMID: 3272814

30. Cheigh JS, Suthanthiran M, Stubenbord WT, et al. Optimization of donor specific blood transfusion in kidney transplantation. Transplant Proc 1987;19:2250-1. PMID: 2978891

31. Chu DZ, Chatterjee SN, Blaisdell FW. A prospective study of pretransplant and operative day blood transfusion on renal allograft recipients. Curr Surg 1982;39:24-6. PMID: 7037317

32. Cochrum K, Hanes D, Potter D, et al. Improved graft survival with donor-specific transfusion pretreatment. Transplant Proc 1981;13:190-3. PMID: 7022820

33. Corry RJ, West JC, Hunsicker LG, et al. Effect of timing of administration and quantity of blood transfusion on cadaver renal transplant survival. Transplantation 1980;30:425-8. PMID: 7008290

34. d'Apice AJ, Sheil AG, Tait BD, et al. A prospective randomized trial of matching for HLA-A and B versus HLA-DR in renal transplantation. Transplantation 1984;38:37-41. PMID: 6377610

35. de Mattos AM, Bennett WM, Barry JM, et al. HLA-identical sibling renal transplantation--a 21-yr single-center experience. Clin Transplant 1999;13:158-67. PMID: 10202612

36. Dewar PJ, Wilkinson R, Elliott RW, et al. Superiority of B locus matching over other HLA matching in renal graft survival. Br Med J (Clin Res Ed) 1982;284:779-82. PMID: 6802225

37. Egidi MF, Scott DH, Corry RJ. The effect of transfusions on renal allograft survival in the cyclosporine era: a single center report. Clin Transplant 1993;7:240-4. PMID: 10148843

38. Eisenberger U, Seifried A, Patey N, et al. FoxP3 positive T cells in graft biopsies from living donor kidney transplants after donor-specific transfusions. Transplantation 2009;87:138-42. PMID: 19136904

39. El-Husseini AA, Foda MA, Shokeir AA, et al. Determinants of graft survival in pediatric and adolescent live donor kidney transplant recipients: a single center experience. Pediatr Transplant 2005;9:763-9. PMID: 16269048

40. Fauchet R, Wattelet J, Genetet B, et al. Role of blood transfusions and pregnancies in kidney transplantation. Vox Sang 1979;37:222-8. PMID: 386612

41. Feduska NJ, Amend WJ, Vincenti F, et al. Graft survival with high levels of cytotoxic antibodies. Transplant Proc 1981;13:73-80. PMID: 7022910

42. Fehrman I. Pretransplant blood transfusions and related kidney allograft survival. Transplantation 1982;34:46-9. PMID: 6214879

43. Fehrman I, Groth CG, Lundgren G, et al. Improved renal graft survival in transfused uremics. A result of a number of interacting factors. Transplantation 1980;30:324-7. PMID: 7006164

44. Flechner SM, Kerman RH, Van Buren C, et al. Successful transplantation of cyclosporine-treated haploidentical living-related renal recipients without blood transfusions. Transplantation 1984;37:73-6. PMID: 6229913

45. Flechner SM, Novick AC, Steinmuller D, et al. Determinants of allograft survival in 100 consecutive cadaver kidney transplants. J Urol 1982;127:1084-6. PMID: 7045404

46. Fonseca HE, Chiba AK, Junior AF, et al. Anti-N-like and anti-Form red cell antibodies in chronic hemodialysis patients. Ren Fail 2004;26:553-6. PMID : 15526914

47. Garcia VD, Kraemer ES, Prompt CA, et al. Donor specific blood transfusions do not improve graft survival in living related donor transplantation. Transplant Proc 1987;19:2271-3. PMID: 3274507

48. Fuller TC, Delmonico FL, Cosimi AB, et al. Effects of virus types of RBC transfusions on HLA alloimmunization and renal allograft survival. Transplant Proc 1977;9:117-9. PMID: 325743

49. Fuller TC, Burroughs JC, Delmonico FL, et al. Influence of frozen blood transfusions on renal allograft survival. Transplant Proc 1982;14:293-5. PMID: 7051469

50. Galvao MM, Peixinho ZF, Mendes NF, et al. Stored blood--an effective immunosuppressive method for transplantation of kidneys from unrelated donors. An 11-year follow-up. Braz J Med Biol Res 1997;30:727-34. PMID: 9292109

51. Garcia LF, Arango AM, Rezonzew R, et al. Donor-specific and random transfusions in HLA-haploidentical kidney transplantation. Transplant Proc 1991;23:1744-6. PMID: 2053141

52. Gardner B, Harris KR, Tate DG, et al. The effect of pretransplant blood transfusions on renal allograft survival in patients on cyclosporine. Transplant Proc 1984;16:1172-3. PMID: 6385368

53. Garvin PJ, Castaneda M, Codd JE, et al. Recipient race as a risk factor in renal transplantation. Arch Surg 1983;118:1441-4. PMID: 6360077

54. Glass NR, Felsheim G, Miller DT, et al. Influence of pre- and perioperative blood transfusions on renal allograft survival. Transplantation 1982;33:430-1. PMID: 7041369

55. Guillou PJ, Will EJ, Davison AM, et al. CAPD--a risk factor in renal transplantation?. Br J Surg 1984;71:878-80. PMID: 6388721

56. Ho-Hsieh H, Novick AC, Steinmuller D, et al. Renal transplantation for end-stage polycystic kidney disease. Urology 1987;30:322-6. PMID: 3310365

57. Hourmant M, Soulillou JP, Bui-Quang D. Beneficial effect of blood transfusion. Role of the time interval between the last transfusion and transplantation. Transplantation 1979;28:40-3. PMID: 377593

58. Hurst PE, Brockis JG, Dawkins RL, et al. Renal transplantation. 12-Year experience. Med J Aust 1981;1:123-6. PMID: 7012562

59. Inoue S, Aikawa M, Dobashi Y, et al. Donor-specific transfusion for kidney transplantation in the cyclosporine era. Transplant Proc 1996;28:1220-1. PMID: 8658633

60. Jakobsen A, Birkeland SA, Gabel H, et al. Renal transplantation in polycystic renal disease--a joint Scandinavian report. Scand J Urol Nephrol Suppl 1980;54:71-5. PMID: 7013048

61. Jeffery JR, Cheung K, Masniuk J, et al. Mixed lymphocyte culture responses. Lack of correlation with cadaveric renal allograft survival and blood transfusions. Transplantation 1984;38:42-5. PMID: 6234685

62. Jeffery JR, Downs A, Grahame JW, et al. Failure of blood transfusions to improve cadaveric renal allograft survival. Transplantation 1978;25:344-5. PMID: 351896

63. Jeffery JR, Downs AR, Grahame JW, et al. Operation-day blood-transfusion and renal transplantation. Lancet 1978;1:662. PMID: 76196

64. Jin DC, Yoon YS, Kim YS, et al. Factors on graft survival of living donor kidney transplantation in a single center. Clin Transplant 1996;10:471-7. PMID: 8996765

65. Jovicic S, Lezaic V, Simonovic R, et al. Beneficial effects of donor-specific transfusion on

renal allograft outcome. Clin Transplant 2010;[Epub ahead of print]: PMID: 20331687

66. Joysey VC, Roger JH, Evans DB, et al. Differential kidney graft survival associated with interaction between recipient ABO group and pretransplant blood transfusion. Transplantation 1977;24:371-6. PMID: 335591

67. Kahn D, Pontin AR, Pike R, et al. The first 100 kidney transplants from living related donors at Groote Schuur Hospital. SAMJ, S Afr med j 1994;84:138-41. PMID: 7740348

68. Kasai I, Kumano K, Iwamura M, et al. Comparative analysis of DST alone and DST with intermittent coverage by cyclophosphamide. Transplant Proc 1989;21:1837-8. PMID: 2652598

69. Kovithavongs T, Schlaut J, Marchuk L, et al. Beneficial effect of blood transfusion in HLA identical and haploidentical renal allografts. Transplant Proc 1982;14:690-2. PMID: 6762727

70. Leivestad T, Albrechtsen D, Flatmark A, et al. Renal transplants from HLA-haploidentical living-related donors. The influence of donor-specific transfusions and different immunosuppressive regimens. Transplantation 1986;42:35-8. PMID: 3523880

71. Lietz K, Lao M, Paczek L, et al. The impact of pretransplant erythropoietin therapy on late outcomes of renal transplantation. Ann Transplant 2003;8:17-24. PMID: 14626572

72. Madsen M, Graugaard B, Fjeldborg O, et al. The impact of HLA-DR antigen matching on the survival of cadaveric renal allografts. A prospective one-center analysis. Transplantation 1983;36:379-83. PMID: 6353704

73. Melzer JS, Husing RM, Feduska NJ, et al. The beneficial effect of pretransplant blood transfusions in cyclosporine-treated cadaver renal allograft recipients. Transplantation 1987;43:61-4. PMID: 3541325

74. Mendez R, Iwaki Y, Mendez R, et al. Effect of deliberate blood transfusions in cadaveric kidney allografts at a single center. J Urol 1982;127:427-9. PMID: 7038148

75. Myburgh JA, Botha JR, Meyers AM, et al. The treatment of end-stage renal disease at the Johannesburg Hospital: a 17-year experience. Part II. The role of transplantation. SAMJ, S Afr med j 1983;64:522-7. PMID: 6353617

76. Norman DJ, Barry JM, Fischer S. The beneficial effect of pretransplant third-party blood transfusions on allograft rejection in HLA-identical sibling kidney transplants. Transplantation 1986;41:125-6. PMID: 3510484

77. Nube MJ, Persijn GG, van Es A, et al. Beneficial effect of HLA-A and B matched pretransplant blood transfusions on primary cadaveric kidney graft survival. Transplantation 1983;35:556-61. PMID: 6346596

78. Oei LS, Thompson JS, Corry RJ. Effect of blood transfusions on survival of cadaver and living related renal transplants. Transplantation 1979;28:482-4. PMID: 390787

79. Okiye SE, Zincke H, Engen DE, et al. Splenectomy in high-risk primary renal transplant recipients. Am J Surg 1983;146:594-601. PMID: 6356949

80. Opelz G, Terasaki PI. Poor kidney-transplant survival in recipients with frozen-blood transfusions or no transfusions. Lancet 1974;2:696-8. PMID: 4142966

81. Persijn GG, van Hooff JP, Kalff MW, et al. Effect of blood transfusions and HLA matching on renal transplantation in the Netherlands. Transplant Proc 1977;9:503-5. PMID: 325789

82. Pfaff WW, Howard RJ, Scornik JC, et al. Incidental and purposeful random donor blood transfusion. Sensitization and transplantation. Transplantation 1989;47:130-3. PMID: 2643223

83. Polesky HF, McCullough JJ, Yunis E, et al. The effects of transfusion of frozen-thawed deglycerolized red cells on renal graft survival. Transplantation 1977;24:449-52. PMID: 339441

84. Poli F, Mascaretti L, Pappalettera M, et al. HLA-DRB1 compatibility in cadaver kidney transplantation: correlation with graft survival and function. Transpl Int 1995;8:91-5. PMID : 7766303

85. Poli L, Pretagostini R, Rossi M, et al. Effect of HLA compatibility, pregnancies, blood transfusions, and taboo mismatches in living unrelated kidney

transplantation. Transplant Proc 2001;33:1136-8. PMID: 11267225

86. Potter DE, Portale AA, Melzer JS, et al. Are blood transfusions beneficial in the cyclosporine era?. Pediatr Nephrol 1991;5:168-72. PMID: 2025530

87. Rao KV, Andersen RC, O'Brien TJ. Factors contributing for improved graft survival in recipients of kidney transplants. Kidney Int 1983;24:210-21. PMID: 6355614

88. Richie RE, Niblack GD, Johnson HK, et al. Factors influencing the outcome of kidney transplants. Ann Surg 1983;197:672-7. PMID : 6344816

89. Sabbaga E, Ianhez LE, Chocair PR, et al. Kidney transplants from living nonrelated donors: an analysis of 87 cases, including 20 cases with specific blood transfusions from the donor. Transplant Proc 1985;17:1741-5. PMID: 3885517

90. Sachs JA, Festenstein H, Tuffnell VA, et al. Collaborative scheme for tissue typing and matching in renal transplantation. IX. Effect of HLA-A, -B, and -D locus matching, pretransplant transfusion, and other factors on 612 cadaver renal grafts. Transplant Proc 1977;9:483-6. PMID: 325785

91. Safwenberg J, Backman-Bave U, Hogman CF. The effect of blood transfusions on cadaver kidney transplants--an analysis of patients transplanted in Uppsala. Scand J Urol Nephrol Suppl 1977;59-61. PMID: 356223

92. Sakagami K, Saito S, Shiozaki S, et al. Renal transplantation from HLA-haploidentical living-related donors: the effects of donor-specific blood transfusions and different immunosuppressive regimens. Acta Med Okayama 1992;46:1-5. PMID: 1561899

93. Salvatierra O,Jr, Melzer J, Vincenti F, et al. Donor-specific blood transfusions versus cyclosporine--the DST story. Transplant Proc 1987;19:160-6. PMID: 3547813

94. Salvatierra O,Jr, Vincenti F, Amend W, et al. Deliberate donor-specific blood transfusions prior to living related renal transplantation. A new approach. Ann Surg 1980;192:543-52. PMID: 6448588

95. Salvatierra O, McVicar J, Melzer J, et al. Improved results with combined donor-specific transfusion (DST) and sequential therapy protocol. Transplant Proc 1991;23:1024-6. PMID: 1989146

96. Sanfilippo F, Thacker L, Vaughn WK. Living-donor renal transplantation in SEOPF. The impact of histocompatibility, transfusions, and cyclosporine on outcome. Transplantation 1990;49:25-9. PMID: 2301022

97. Sells RA, Scott MH, Prieto M, et al. Early rejection following donor-specific transfusion prior to HLA-mismatched living related renal transplantation. Transplant Proc 1989;21:1173-4. PMID: 2650088

98. Sengar DP, Rashid A, Jindal SL. Effect of blood transfusions on renal allograft survival. Transplant Proc 1979;11:179-81. PMID: 377627

99. Sijpkens YW, Koep LJ, Persijn GG, et al. Pros and cons of donor-specific blood transfusions in living related kidney transplantation. Neth J Med 1984;27:1-5. PMID: 6231486

100. Sirchia G, Mercuriali F, Pizzi C, et al. Blood transfusion and kidney transplantation: effect of small doses of blood on kidney graft function and survival. Transplant Proc 1982;14:263-71. PMID : 7051464

101. Sirchia G, Mercuriali F, Scalamogna M, et al. Evaluation of the blood transfusion policy of the north Italy transplant program. Transplantation 1981;31:388-94. PMID: 7015627

102. Solheim BG, Flatmark A, Halvorsen S, et al. The effect of blood transfusions on renal transplantation. Studies of 395 patients registered for transplantation with a first cadaveric kidney. Tissue Antigens 1980;16:377-86. PMID: 7008257

103. Solheim BG, Flatmark A, Halvorsen S, et al. Effect of blood transfusions on renal transplantation: study of 191 consecutive first transplants from living related donors. Transplantation 1980;30:281-4. PMID: 6449767

104. Sommer BG, Ferguson RM. Mismatched living, related donor renal transplantation: a prospective, randomized study. Surgery 1985;98:267-74. PMID: 3895539

105. Spees EK, Vaughn WK, McDonald JC, et al. Why do secondary cadaver renal transplants succeed? Results of the South-Eastern Organ Procurement

Foundation prospective study, 1977-1982. J Urol 1983;129:484-8. PMID: 6339749

106. Spees EK, Vaughn WK, Williams GM, et al. Effects of blood transfusion on cadaver renal transplantation: the Southeastern Organ Procurement Foundation prospective study (1977 to 1979). Transplantation 1980;30:455-63. PMID: 7008295

107. Stiller CR, Lockwood BL, Sinclair NR, et al. Beneficial effect of operation-day blood-transfusions on human renal-allograft survival. Lancet 1978;1:169-70. PMID: 74601

108. Takahashi I, Otsubo O, Nishimura M, et al. Prolonged graft survival by donor-specific blood transfusion (DSBT). Transplant Proc 1982;14:367-9. PMID: 7051481

109. Takiff H, Cook DJ, Himaya NS, et al. Dominant effect of histocompatibility on ten-year kidney transplant survival. Transplantation 1988;45:410-5. PMID: 3278435

110. Thorsby E, Moen T, Solheim BG, et al. Influence of HLA matching in cadaveric renal transplantation: experience from one Scandiatransplant center. Tissue Antigens 1981;17:83-90. PMID: 7018015

111. Ting A, Morris PJ. The influence of HLA-A,B and -DR matching and pregraft blood transfusions on graft and patient survival after renal transplantation in a single centre. Tissue Antigens 1984;24:256-64. PMID: 6393428

112. Velidedeoglu E, Tokyay R, Haberal M. Effect of donor-specific blood transfusions on graft outcome in live donor renal transplantations. Transplant Proc 1992;24:2752-3. PMID: 1465927

113. Waanders MM, Roelen DL, de Fijter JW, et al. Protocolled blood transfusions in recipients of a simultaneous pancreas-kidney transplant reduce severe acute graft rejection. Transplantation 2008;85:1668-70. PMID: 18551077

114. Walker JF, Oreopoulos DG, Uldall PR, et al. The effect of pre-transplant blood transfusion on graft outcome in patients on peritoneal dialysis prior to renal transplantation. Transplant Proc 1982;14:687-9. PMID: 6762726

115. Walter S, Poulsen LR, Friedberg M, et al. The effect of blood-transfusions on renal allograft survival. Scand J Urol Nephrol Suppl 1977;62-4. PMID: 356225

116. Werner-Favre C, Jeannet M, Harder F, et al. Blood transfusions, cytotoxic antibodies, and kidney graft survival. Preliminary results of a systematic transfusion protocol. Transplantation 1979;28:343-6. PMID: 388766

117. Xiao X, Li Y, Ao J, et al. Analysis of prognostic factors affecting renal allograft survival. Transpl Int 1992;5:226-30. PMID: 1418314

118. Yamauchi J, Akiyama N, Sugimoto H, et al. Uselessness of donor-specific transfusions or prophylactic ALG with therapeutic cyclosporine doses in living related renal transplantation between one-haplotype matched pairs. Transplant Proc 1989;21:1663-6. PMID: 2652545

119. Zeichner WD, Toledo-Pereyra LH, Whitten J, et al. Lack of correlation between cadaver kidney transplant survival and the number of pretransplant transfusions. Transplantation 1983;35:500-1. PMID: 6342229

120. Frisk B, Brynger H, Sandberg L. Two random transfusions before primary renal transplantation--four years' experience from a single center. Transplant Proc 1982;14:386-8. PMID: 7051484

121. Solheim BG, Flatmark A, Halvorsen S, et al. Effect of pre-transplant blood transfusions and haemodialysis on the survival of first kidney grafts from living related donors. Scand J Urol Nephrol Suppl 1980;54:63-6. PMID: 7013047

122. Reed A, Pirsch J, Armbrust MJ, et al. Multivariate analysis of donor-specific versus random transfusion protocols in haploidentical living-related transplants. Transplantation 1991;51:382-4. PMID: 1994532

123. Sanfilippo F, Vaughn WK, LeFor WM, et al. Multivariate analysis of risk factors in cadaver donor kidney transplantation. Transplantation 1986;42:28-34. PMID: 3523879

124. Tang H, Chelamcharla M, Baird BC, et al. Factors affecting kidney-transplant outcome in recipients with lupus nephritis. Clin Transplant 2008;22:263-72. PMID: 18482047

125. Peters TG, Shaver TR, Ames JE,4th, et al. Cold ischemia and outcome in 17,937 cadaveric kidney transplants. Transplantation 1995;59:191-6. PMID: 7839440

126. Sautner T, Gruenberger T, Barlan M, et al. Immunological risk factors are solely responsible for primary non-function of renal allografts. Transpl Int 1994;7:S294-7. PMID: 11271229

127. Madrenas J, Newman S, McGregor JR, et al. An alternative approach for statistical analysis of kidney transplant data: multivariate analysis of single-center experience. Am J Kidney Dis 1988;12:524-30. PMID: 3057883

128. A randomized clinical trial of cyclosporine in cadaveric renal transplantation. Analysis at three years. The Canadian multicentre transplant study group. N Engl J Med 1986;314:1219-25. PMID: 2871486

129. Nube MJ, Persijn GG, Kalff MW, et al. Transplant survival and clinical course after pretransplant HLA-A and B matched blood transfusions: a single centre study. Proc Eur Dial Transplant Assoc 1983;19:445-52. PMID: 6348745

130. Brynger H, Frisk B, Ahlmen J, et al. Blood transfusion and primary graft survival in male recipients. Scand J Urol Nephrol Suppl 1977;76-8. PMID: 356229

131. Akiyama N, Otsubo O, Yamauchi J, et al. Effects of donor-specific blood transfusion on the survival of living related renal grafts. Jpn J Exp Med 1984;54:225-7. PMID: 6398837

132. Huprikar AG, Arora N, Bulchand S. Donor specific transfusions in renal transplantation. J Assoc Physicians India 1987;35:577-9. PMID: 3320025

133. Glass NR, Miller DT, Sollinger HW, et al. A four-year experience with donor blood transfusion protocols for living-donor renal transplantation. Transplantation 1985;39:615-9. PMID: 3890291

134. Padanyi A, Horuzsko A, Gyodi E, et al. Long-term related kidney graft survival in high-risk patients after monitored donor-specific transfusion protocol. Transpl Int 1998;11:S110-4. PMID: 9664958

135. Takahashi K, Yagisawa T, Tanabe I, et al. Outcome of kidney transplantation in highly sensitized patients after donor-specific blood transfusion. Transplant Proc 1987;19:3655-60. PMID: 2960043

136. Casadei DH, Cambariere R, Leanza H, et al. Donor specific blood transfusion in renal transplantation: analysis of 22 cases. Transplant Proc 1987;19:2274-5. PMID: 3079079

137. Andrus CH, Betts RF, May AG, et al. Cytomegalovirus infection blocks the beneficial effect of pretransplant blood transfusion on renal allograft survival. Transplantation 1979;28:451-6. PMID: 229593

138. Chavers BM, Sullivan EK, Tejani A, et al. Pre-transplant blood transfusion and renal allograft outcome: a report of the North American Pediatric Renal Transplant Cooperative Study. Pediatr Transplant 1997;1:22-8. PMID : 10084783

139. Fradet Y, Roy R, Lachance JG, et al. Kidney graft survival: role of blood transfusions and lymphocytotoxic antibodies. Clin Nephrol 1982;18:69-73. PMID: 6754190

140. Husberg B, Lindergard B, Lindholm T, et al. Blood transfusion and kidney transplantation. Scand J Urol Nephrol Suppl 1977;73-5. PMID: 356228

141. Kerman RH, Kimball PM, Van Buren CT, et al. Possible contribution of pretransplant immune responder status to renal allograft survival differences of black versus white recipients. Transplantation 1991;51:338-42. PMID: 1825242

142. Kerman RH, Van Buren CT, Lewis RM, et al. Impact of blood transfusions and HLA on cyclosporine-treated renal transplant recipients. Transplant Proc 1988;20:264-9. PMID: 3291254

143. Kerman RH, Van Buren CT, Payne W, et al. The influence on pretransplant blood transfusions from random donors on immune parameters affecting cadaveric allograft survival. Transplantation 1983;36:50-4. PMID: 6223421

144. Muller GA, Muller C, Bockhorn H, et al. HLA-DR-MT matching improves graft survival rate in cadaver kidney transplantation. A prospective multicenter analysis of the South German Cooperative Study Group for Kidney Transplantation. Klin Wochenschr 1983;61:17-23. PMID: 6187967

145. van Es A, Persijn GG, van Hooff-Eijkenboom YE, et al. Blood transfusions, HLA-A and B, DR matching, graft survival, and clinical course after cadaveric kidney transplantation. Transplant Proc 1981;13:172-4. PMID: 7022816

146. Velasco N, Catto GR, Edward N, et al. The effect of the dosage of steroids on the incidence of cytomegalovirus infections in renal transplant recipients. J Infect 1984;9:69-78. PMID: 6094670

147. Perkins HA, Salvatierra O. Correlation of renal allograft survival with previous blood transfusions. Transplant Proc 1977;9:209-10. PMID: 324050

148. Cheigh JS, Saal SD, Suthanthiran M, et al. Natural history of cadaveric kidney transplants in the absence of early acute rejection. Nephron 1983;35:6-10. PMID: 6193438

149. Cho SI, Bradley JW, Carpenter CB, et al. Antithymocyte globulin, pretransplant blood transfusion, and tissue typing in cadaver kidney transplantation. Am J Surg 1983;145:464-71. PMID: 6340551

150. Vathsala A, Tan S, Woo KT, et al. The impact of HLA match transfusions and presensitization on renal transplantation in the cyclosporine era. Ann Acad Med Singapore 1992;21:364-7. PMID: 1416786

151. Higgins RM, Raymond NT, Krishnan NS, et al. Acute rejection after renal transplantation is reduced by approximately 50% by prior therapeutic blood transfusions, even in tacrolimus-treated patients. Transplantation 2004;77:469-71. PMID: 14966430

152. Park YH, Min SK, Lee JN, et al. Risk factors on graft survival of living donor kidney transplantation. Transplant Proc 2004;36:2023-5. PMID: 15518732

153. Bunnapradist S, Daswani A, Takemoto SK. Graft survival following living-donor renal transplantation: a comparison of tacrolimus and cyclosporine microemulsion with mycophenolate mofetil and steroids. Transplantation 2003;76:10-5. PMID: 12865780

154. Agarwal SK, Dash SC, Mehta SN, et al. Results of renal transplantation on conventional immunosuppression in second decade in India: a single centre experience. J Assoc Physicians India 2002;50:532-6. PMID : 12164404

155. Montagnino G, Tarantino A, Maccario M, et al. Long-term results with cyclosporine monotherapy in renal transplant patients: a multivariate analysis of risk factors. Am J Kidney Dis 2000;35:1135-43. PMID: 10845828

156. Herget-Rosenthal S, Gerken G, Philipp T, et al. Serum ferritin and survival of renal transplant recipients: a prospective 10-year cohort study. Transpl Int 2003;16:642-7. PMID: 12732929

157. Sanfilippo FP, Bollinger RR, MacQueen JM, et al. A randomized study comparing leukocyte-depleted versus packed red cell transfusions in prospective cadaver renal allograft recipients. Transfusion 1985;25:116-9. PMID: 3885483

158. Persijn GG, van Leeuwen A, Parlevliet J, et al. Two major factors influencing kidney graft survival in Eurotransplant: HLA-DR matching and blood transfusion(s). Transplant Proc 1981;13:150-4. PMID: 7022812

159. Cecka JM. Calculated PRA (CPRA): the new measure of sensitization for transplant candidates. Am J Transplantation 2010;10:26-9. PMID: 19958328

160. Hajeer AH. Panel reactive antibody test (PRA) in renal transplantation. Saudi J Kidney Dis Transplant 2006;17:1-4. PMID: 17297529

161. Worthington JE, Robson AJ, Sheldon S, et al. A comparison of enzyme-linked immunoabsorbent assays and flow cytometry techniques for the detection of HLA specific antibodies. Hum Immunol 2001;62:1178-84. PMID: 11600227

162. Harmer AW, Heads AJ, Vaughan RW. Detection of HLA class I and class II specific antibodies by flow cytometry and PRA-Stat screening in renal transplant recipients. Transplantation 1997;63:1828-32. PMID: 9210512

163. Buelow R, Mercier I, Glanville L, et al. Detection of panel-reactive anti-HLA class I antibodies by enzyme-linked immunosorbent assay or lymphcytotoxicity: results of a blinded, controlled multicenter study. Hum Immunol 1995;44:1-11. PMID: 8522449

164. Kerman RH, Susskind B, Beulow R, et al. Correlation of ELISA-detected igG and IgA anti-HLA antibodies in pretransplant sera with renal allograft rejection. Transplantation 1996;62:201-5. PMID: 8755816

165. Bryan CF, Baier KA, Flora-Ginter G, et al. Detection of HLA IgG antibodies by two enzyme-linked immunoassays, solubilized HLA class I and PRA-STAT: comparison with the AHG PRA. Transplantation 1995;6260:1588-94. PMID: 8545895

166. Vieira CA, Agarwal A., Book BK, et al. Rituximab for reduction of anti-HLA antibodies in patients awaiting renal transplantation: safety, pharmacodynamics, and pharmacokinetics. Transplantation 2004;77:542-8. PMID: 15084932

167. Vo A.A., Lukovsky M, Wang J, et al. Rituximab and intravenous immune globulin for desensitization during renal transplantation. N Engl J Med 2008;359:242-51. PMID: 18635429

168. Muhmoud KM, Sobh MA, el Shenawy F, et al. Management of sensitized patients awaiting renal transplantation: does sequential therapy with intravenous immunoglobulin and simvastatin offer a solution. Eur J Cancer Clin Oncol 2007;56:202-5. PMID: 17296177

169. Nurhan-Ozdemir F, Akcay A, Sezer S, et al. Effect of simvastatin in the treatment of highly sensitized dialysis patients: the pre and post-renal transplantation follow-up outcomes. Transplant immunology 2004;13:39-42. PMID: 15203127

170. Alarabi A, Backman-Bave U, Wikstrom B, et al. Plasmapheresis in HLA-immunosensitized patients prior to kidney transplantation. Int J Artificial Organs 1997;201:51-6. PMID: 9062832

171. Akcay A, Ozdemir FN, Atac FB, et al. Angiotensin-Converting Enzyme genotype is a predictive factor in the peak panel-reactive antibody response. Transplant Proc 2004;36:35-7. PMID: 15013293

172. Buscaroli A, nanni-Costa A, Iannelli Sea. Value of panel reactive antibodies (PRA) as a guide to the treatment of hyperimmunized patients in renal transplant. Transpl Int 1992;5(Suppl 1):s54-7. PMID: 14621731

173. d'Apice AJ, Tait BD. An elective transfusion policy: sensitization rates, patient transplantability, and transplant outcome. Transplantation 1982;33:191-5. PMID: 7036472

174. Opelz G, Mickey MR, Terasaki PI. Responsiveness to HL-A as studied by monitoring blood transfusions and kidney transplants. Proc Eur Dial Transplant Assoc 1973;10:471-4. PMID: 4607029

175. Albrechtsen D, Flatmark A, Lundgren G, et al. Renal transplantation from HLA-haploidentical living related donors: the Scandinavian multicenter study of the effects of cyclosporine immunosuppression. Clinical transplantation 1987;1:104-7.

176. Opelz G, Terasaki P. Histocompatibility matching utilizing responsiveness as a new dimension. TRANSPLANT-PROC 1972;4:433-7. PMID: 4566783

177. Opelz G, Collaborative Transplant Study. Non-HLA transplantation immunity revealed by lymphocytotoxic antibodies. Lancet 2005;365:1570-6. PMID: 15866311

178. Terasaki PI, Perdue ST, Sasaki N, et al. Improving success rates of kidney transplantation. JAMA 1983;250:1065-8. PMID: 6348321

Appendix A. Ovid MEDLINE Search Strategy

1. Kidney Transplantation/ (68861)
2. (kidney adj2 transplant$).mp. [mp=title, original title, abstract, name of substance word, subject heading word, unique identifier] (71289)
3. (renal adj2 transplant$).mp. [mp=title, original title, abstract, name of substance word, subject heading word, unique identifier] (32401)
4. (kidney adj2 allograft$).mp. [mp=title, original title, abstract, name of substance word, subject heading word, unique identifier] (2226)
5. (renal adj2 allograft$).mp. [mp=title, original title, abstract, name of substance word, subject heading word, unique identifier] (9486)
6. (kidney adj3 recipient$).mp. [mp=title, original title, abstract, name of substance word, subject heading word, unique identifier] (5604)
7. (renal adj3 recipient$).mp. [mp=title, original title, abstract, name of substance word, subject heading word, unique identifier] (11515)
8. kidney graft$.mp. (2474)
9. renal graft$.mp. (2074)
10. 1 or 2 or 3 or 4 or 5 or 6 or 7 or 8 or 9 (76294)
11. erythrocyte transfusion$.mp. or Erythrocyte Transfusion/ (5064)
12. ((donor specific adj2 transfusion$) or DST).mp. [mp=title, original title, abstract, name of substance word, subject heading word, unique identifier] (2700)
13. ((pretransplant adj2 transfusion$) or PTF).mp. [mp=title, original title, abstract, name of substance word, subject heading word, unique identifier] (596)
14. ((red adj2 cell transfusion$) or RBC transfusion$).mp. [mp=title, original title, abstract, name of substance word, subject heading word, unique identifier] (2547)
15. ((random adj3 transfusion$) or rPTF).mp. [mp=title, original title, abstract, name of substance word, subject heading word, unique identifier] (164)
16. ((matched adj3 transfusion$) or mPTF).mp. [mp=title, original title, abstract, name of substance word, subject heading word, unique identifier] (175)
17. blood transfusion$.tw. (24574)
18. 11 or 12 or 13 or 14 or 15 or 16 or 17 (33059)
19. 10 and 18 (1421)
20. limit 19 to humans (1276)
21. limit 20 to "review articles" (94)
22. 20 not 21 (1182)

Appendix B. Embase Search Strategy

No.	Query	Results
#23	#21 NOT #20 AND ([controlled clinical trial]/lim OR [randomized controlled trial]/lim) AND [embase]/lim	7
#22	#21 NOT #20	390
#21	#11 AND #18 AND [humans]/lim	7480
#20	#11 AND #18 AND [humans]/lim AND [english]/lim AND [embase]/lim	7090
#19	#11 AND #18	9010
#18	#12 OR #13 OR #14 OR #15 OR #16 OR #17	143022
#17	random AND ('transfusion'/exp OR transfusion) AND [embase]/lim	1212
#16	'donor'/exp OR donor AND specific AND ('transfusion'/exp OR transfusion) AND [embase]/lim	4032
#15	pretransplant AND ('transfusion'/exp OR transfusion) AND [embase]/lim	1099
#14	red AND ('blood'/exp OR blood) AND ('cell'/exp OR cell) AND ('transfusion'/exp OR transfusion) AND [embase]/lim	14227
#13	'blood'/exp OR blood AND ('transfusion'/exp OR transfusion) AND [embase]/lim	140653
#12	'erythrocyte'/exp OR erythrocyte AND ('transfusion'/exp OR transfusion) AND [embase]/lim	38988
#11	#1 OR #2 OR #3 OR #4 OR #5 OR #6 OR #7 OR #8 OR #9 OR #10	124632
#10	renal AND recipients AND [embase]/lim	19546
#9	'kidney'/exp OR kidney AND recipients AND [embase]/lim	24190
#8	renal AND graft AND [embase]/lim	42244
#7	'kidney'/exp OR kidney AND graft AND [embase]/lim	54612
#6	renal AND ('allograft'/exp OR allograft) AND [embase]/lim	14954
#5	'kidney'/exp OR kidney AND ('allograft'/exp OR allograft) AND [embase]/lim	17271
#4	renal AND transplant AND [embase]/lim	52527
#3	'kidney'/exp OR kidney AND transplant AND [embase]/lim	66160
#2	renal AND ('transplantation'/exp OR transplantation) AND [embase]/lim	80779
#1	'kidney'/exp OR kidney AND ('transplantation'/exp OR transplantation) AND [embase]/lim	108266

Appendix C. Demographics Table

Characteristics of Unique Studies Included for Evaluations

Study, Year (N=)	Study Design	Study Period	Population	Transfusion type* Exp (%) Control (%)	Type of control groups	Accounted for confounding	Demographic data in both groups[†]	Validity of the study
Jovicic S, 2010 (N=159)	ROBS	1990-2000	Patients receiving living donor renal transplants	DST (9) RBT (83) NT (8)	Concurrent	Yes	Yes	Fair
Aalten J, 2009 (N=859)	ROBS	1996-2006	Female patients receiving primary renal transplants	DST (6) PT (8) RBT (42) NT (44)	Concurrent	Yes	Yes	Fair
Eisenberger U, 2009 (N=138)	ROBS	1990-2005	Patients receiving living donor renal transplants	DST (50) NT (50)	Historical	No	Yes	Poor
Tang H, 2008 (N=2,882)	ROBS	1995-2002	Patients with ESRD caused by SLE undergoing renal transplant	RBT (63) NT (37)	Concurrent	Yes	No	Poor
Waanders MM, 2008 (N=118)	ROBS	1996-2005	Patients receiving simultaneous pancreas-renal transplants	PT (42) NT (58)	Concurrent	Yes	Yes	Fair
Marti HP, 2006 (N=110)	CCT	1993-2003	Patients receiving living renal transplants	DST (50) NT (50)	Concurrent	Yes	Yes	Good
El-Husseini AA, 2005 (N=284)	ROBS	1976-2004	Patients (≤ 20 years) receiving living donor renal transplants	RBT (58) NT (42)	Concurrent	Yes	No	Poor
Opelz G, 2005 (N= 164,534)	ROBS	1982-2002	Patients receiving renal transplants, who were included in the international Collaborative Transplant Study	NR	Concurrent	Yes	No	Poor
Higgins RM, 2004 (N=265)	ROBS	1994-2002	Patients receiving renal transplants, treated with CyA or Tac	RBT ≥ 3 (54) RBT 0-2 (46)[‡]	Concurrent	Yes	No	Poor

Study, Year (N=)	Study Design	Study Period	Population	Transfusion type* Exp (%) Control (%)	Type of control groups	Accounted for confounding	Demographic data in both groups†	Validity of the study
Park YH, 2004 (N=77)	ROBS	1991-2003	Patients receiving living-related renal transplants	RBT (18) NT (82)	Concurrent	Yes	No	Poor
Bunnapradist S, 2003 (N=7079)	ROBS	1988-1999	Patients receiving cadaver renal transplants, treated with CyA-MMF or Tac-MMF	NR	Concurrent	Yes	Yes	Fair
Herget-Rosenthal S, 2003 (N=NR)	POBS	1990-NR	Renal transplant recipients with serum ferritin levels above 1,100 ng/mL	NR	Concurrent	Yes	No	Poor
Lietz K, 2003 (N=267)	ROBS	1990-1997	Patients receiving renal transplants whose graft survived > 6 months	RBT (78) NT (22)	Concurrent	Yes	No	Poor
Agarwal SK, 2002 (N=144)	ROBS	1980-1989	Patients receiving living-related renal transplants	NR	Concurrent	Yes	No	Poor
Barbari A, 2001 (N=84)	ROBS	NR	Patients receiving renal transplants	DST (76) NT (24)	Concurrent	No	No	Poor
Hiesse C, 2001 (N=106)	CCT	1992-1996	Transfusion naïve cadaverrenal transplant recipients	PT (66) NT (34)	Concurrent	Yes	Yes	Good
Poli L, 2001 (N=514)	ROBS	1967-2000	Patients receiving living donor renal transplants	RBT (43) NT (57)	Concurrent	No	No	Poor
Montagnino G, 2000 (N=143)	Pooled analysis of CCT	NR	Patients receiving primary renal transplants	NR	NR	Yes	No	Poor
Alexander JW, 1999 (N=212)	CCT	1992-1996	Patients receiving non-HLA identical living renal transplants	DST (54) NT (46)	Concurrent	Yes	Yes	Good
de Mattos AM, 1999 (N=107)	ROBS	1977-1993	Patients receiving HLA-identical sibling renal transplants	RBT (79) NT (21)	Concurrent	No	No	Poor

Study, Year (N=)	Study Design	Study Period	Population	Transfusion type* Exp (%) Control (%)	Type of control groups	Accounted for confounding	Demographic data in both groups†	Validity of the study
Padányi A, 1998 (N=57)	ROBS	NR	Patients receiving living-related renal transplants	DST (23) RBT (77)	Concurrent	No	No	Poor
Chavers BM, 1997 (N=4015)	ROBS	1987-1995	Pediatric patients (<18 years old) receiving renal transplants	RBT (71) NT (29)	Concurrent	No	No	Poor
Galvao M, 1997 (N=60)	ROBS	1983-NR	Patients receiving living, unrelated renal transplants	DST (62) NT (38)	Concurrent	No	Yes	Poor
Opelz G, 1997 (N=423)	CCT	1987-1994	Patients receiving primary cadaver renal transplants	RBT (48) NT (52)	Concurrent	Yes	Yes	Good
Sharma RK, 1997 (N=30)	CCT	1992-1993	Patients receiving living-related renal transplants	DST (50) NT (50)	Concurrent	Yes	Yes	Good
Inoue S, 1996 (N=115)	ROBS	1982-1993	Patients receiving living donor renal transplants	DST (37) NT (63)	Concurrent	Yes	No	Poor
Jin DC, 1996 (N=680)	ROBS	1969-1994	Patients receiving primary living-donor transplants, treated with CyA	DST (22) NT (78)	Concurrent	Yes	No	Poor
Peters TG, 1995 (N=17,937)	ROBS	1982-1991	Patients receiving cadaver renal transplants	RBT (NR) NT (NR)	NR	Yes	No	Poor
Poli F, 1995 (N=416)	ROBS	1989-1993	Patients receiving cadaver renal transplants	RBT (51) NT (49)	Concurrent	Yes	No	Poor
Barber WH, 1994 (N=598)	ROBS	1981-1987	Patients receiving one-haplotype matched living-related renal transplants	DST (48) NT (52)	Concurrent	No	No	Poor
Kahn D, 1994 (N=49)	ROBS	1970-1988	Patients receiving 1-haplotype matched, living-related renal transplants	DST (61) NT (39)	Concurrent	No	No	Poor
Sautner T, 1994 (N=73)	ROBS	1982-1991	Grafts with primary non-function, with data required from both kidneys of each donor	RBT (81) NT (19)	Concurrent	Yes	No	Poor

Study, Year (N=)	Study Design	Study Period	Population	Transfusion type* Exp (%) Control (%)	Type of control groups	Accounted for confounding	Demographic data in both groups†	Validity of the study
Egidi MF, 1993 (N=248)	ROBS	1984-1990	Patients receiving primary renal transplants, treated with CyA	RBT (83) NT (17)	Concurrent	No	Yes	Poor
Basri N, 1992 (N=53)	POBS	1988-1990	Patients receiving haploidentical living-related renal transplants	DST (53) NT (47)	Concurrent	No	No	Poor
Sakagami K, 1992 (N=109)	ROBS	1974-1991	Patients receiving haploidentical living-related donor renal transplants	DST (49) NT (51)	Concurrent	No	Yes	Poor
Vathsala A, 1992 (N=116)	ROBS	1984-1990	Patients receiving cadaver renal transplants	RBT >7 (37) RBT <7 (63)‡	Concurrent	No	Yes	Poor
Velidedeoglu E, 1992 (N=437)	ROBS	1985-1990	Patients receiving ABO-compatible, living donor renal transplants	DST (79) NT (21)	Concurrent	Yes	Yes	Fair
Xiao X, 1992 (N=201)	ROBS	1977-1990	Patients receiving cadaver renal transplants	RBT (76) NT (23)	Concurrent	No	No	Poor
Garcia LF, 1991 (N=NR)	ROBS	1982-NR	Patients receiving haploidentical living-related donor renal transplants	DST (n=NR) RBT(n=NR) NT (n=13)	Historical	No	No	Poor
Kerman RH, 1991 (N=324)	ROBS	NR	Patients receiving primary cadaver renal transplants, treated with CyA	RBT (62) NT (38)	Concurrent	No	No	Poor
Potter DE, 1991 (N=634)	ROBS	1983-1989	Patients (adults and children) receiving primary cadaver renal transplants	RBT (71) NT (29)	Concurrent	No	No	Poor
Reed A, 1991 (N=119)	ROBS	1986-1989	Patients receiving living-related renal transplants	DST (56) RBT (44)	Concurrent	Yes	Yes	Fair
Salvatierra O, 1991 (N=118)	ROBS	1986-1990	Patients with 1- and 2-haplotype mismatches with living donor renal transplants	DST (60) NT (40)	Concurrent	No	No	Poor
Sanfilippo F, 1990 (N=2138)	POBS	1983-1988	Patients receiving primary living donor renal transplants	DST (68) NT (32)	Concurrent	No	No	Poor

Study, Year (N=)	Study Design	Study Period	Population	Transfusion type* Exp (%) Control (%)	Type of control groups	Accounted for confounding	Demographic data in both groups†	Validity of the study
Kasai I, 1989 (N=26)	ROBS	NR	Patients receiving living-related renal transplants	DST (73) NT (27)	Concurrent	No	No	Poor
Pfaff WW, 1989 (N=392)	POBS	1980-1987	Patients receiving primary renal transplant	PT (83) NT (17)	Concurrent	No	No	Poor
Sells RA, 1989 (N=134)	ROBS	NR	Patients receiving HLA mismatched living-related renal transplants	DST (60) NT (40)	Concurrent	No	No	Poor
Yamauchi J, 1989 (N=28)	ROBS	1984-1988	Patients receiving HLA haploidentical living-related renal transplants	DST (68) NT (32)	Concurrent	No	No	Poor
Albrechtsen D, 1988 (N=701)	CCT	1982-1985	Patients receiving renal transplants	RBT (68) NT (32)	Concurrent	No	Yes	Fair
Brynger H, 1988 (N=459)	CCT	1985-1987	Patients receiving primary cadaver renal transplants	RBT (63) NT (37)	Concurrent	No	No	Poor
Bucin D, 1988 (N=116)	ROBS	1979-1982	Patients receiving renal transplants	RBT (68) NT (32)	Concurrent	No	Yes	Poor
Kerman RH, 1988 (N=320)	ROBS	NR	Patients receiving primary cadaveric renal transplants	RBT (69) NT (31)	Concurrent	No	No	Poor
Madrenas J, 1988 (N=287)	ROBS	1975-1985	Patients receiving renal transplants	RBT (81) NT (19)	Concurrent	Yes	No	Poor
Takiff H, 1988 (N=NR)	ROBS	1974-1986	Patients receiving primary cadaveric renal transplants	RBT (NR) NT (NR)	Concurrent	No	No	Fair§
Alarif 1987 (N=121)	ROBS	1984-1985	Patients receiving renal transplants	RBT (100)	NR	No	No	Poor
Casadei DH, 1987 (N=42)	ROBS	1978-1985	Patients receiving haploidentical or histoidentical renal transplants	DST+RBT (52) RBT (48)	Historical	No	No	Poor

Study, Year (N=)	Study Design	Study Period	Population	Transfusion type* Exp (%) Control (%)	Type of control groups	Accounted for confounding	Demographic data in both groups[†]	Validity of the study
Cheigh JS, 1987 (N=90)	POBS	NR	Patients receiving one-haplotype mismatched living-related renal transplants	DST (44) NT (56)	Historical	No	No	Poor
Garcia VD, 1987 (N=89)	ROBS	1982-1986	Patients receiving living-donor renal transplants	DST (39) NT (61)	Concurrent	No	Yes	Poor
Ho-Hsieh H, 1987 (N=51)	ROBS	1963-1984	Patients with ADPKD receiving renal transplants	RBT (65) NT (35)	Historical	No	No	Poor
Huprikar AG, 1987 (N=66)	ROBS	1983-1986	Patients (age=12-60 years) receiving primary renal transplants	DST (50) RBT (50)	Concurrent	No	No	Poor
Melzer JS, 1987 (N=212)	ROBS	1983-1985	Patients receiving primary cadaver renal transplants	RBT (77) NT (23)	Concurrent	No	Yes	Poor
Salvatierra O, 1987 (N=230)	ROBS	1978-1986	Patients receiving HLA-identical renal transplants	DST (17) NT (83)	Concurrent	No	No	Poor
Takahashi K, 1987 (N=290)	ROBS	1983-1987	Patients receiving living-related renal transplants	DST (59) RBT (41)	Concurrent	No	No	Poor
Leivestad T, 1986 (N=74)	ROBS	1980-1984	Potential primary graft recipients of a haploidentical living-related renal transplant	DST (43) NT (57)	Concurrent	No	No	Poor
CMTSG, 1986 (N=291)	CCT	1980-1985	Patients receiving cadaveric renal transplants	NR	Concurrent	Yes	No	Fair
Norman DJ, 1986 (N=43)	ROBS	1980-1984	Patients receiving HLA-identical sibling renal transplants	RBT (58) NT (42)	Concurrent	No	No	Poor
Sanfilippo F, 1986 (N=3,628)	ROBS	1977-1982	Patients receiving cadaver renal transplants	RBT (NR) NT (NR)	NR	Yes	No	Poor

Study, Year (N=)	Study Design	Study Period	Population	Transfusion type* Exp (%) Control (%)	Type of control groups	Accounted for confounding	Demographic data in both groups†	Validity of the study
Glass NR, 1985 (N=206)	ROBS	1980-1984	Patients receiving living-donor transplants	DST (64) RBT (36)	Concurrent	No	Yes	Poor
Sabbaga E, 1985 (N=40)	ROBS	1971-1983	Patients receiving living non-related donor transplants	DST (50) NT (50)	Concurrent	No	Yes	Poor
Sanfilippo F, 1985 (N=87)	CCT	1980-1982	Potential candidates for cadaver renal transplants	LT (52) RBT (48)	Concurrent	Yes	No	Poor
Sommer BG, 1985 (N=27)	CCT	NR	Patients receiving living-related renal transplants	DST (37) NT (63)	Concurrent	Yes	Yes	Fair
Akiyama N, 1984 (N=19)	ROBS	1977-1982	Patients receiving 1-haplotype mismatched living-related renal transplants	DST (58) RBT (42)	Concurrent	No	No	Poor
d'Apice AJ, 1984 (N=337)	CCT	1979-1981	Patients receiving renal transplants	RBT (83) NT (17)	Concurrent	Yes	No	Fair
Flechner SM, 1984 (N=36)	ROBS	1981-1983	Patients receiving haplotype-matched living-related renal transplants	RBT (58) NT (42)	Historical	No	No	Poor
Gardner B, 1984 (N=100)	ROBS	NR	Patients receiving renal transplants, treated with CyA	RBT (75) NT (25)	Concurrent	No	No	Poor
Guillou PJ, 1984 (N=114)	ROBS	1981-1984	Patients receiving cadaver renal transplants	RBT(56) NT (44)	Concurrent	No	Yes	Poor
Jeffery JR, 1984 (N=NR)	ROBS	1975-1979?	Patients receiving renal transplants	RBT (NR) NT (NR)	Concurrent	No	No	Poor
Sijpkens YWJ, 1984 (N=59)	POBS	1979-1981	Patients receiving living-related renal transplants	DST (56) NT (44)	Historical	No	Yes	Fair

Study, Year (N=)	Study Design	Study Period	Population	Transfusion type* Exp (%) Control (%)	Type of control groups	Accounted for confounding	Demographic data in both groups†	Validity of the study
Ting A, 1984 (N=298)	ROBS	1975-1983	Patients receiving primary cadaver renal transplant	RBT (57) NT (43)	Concurrent	No	No	Poor
Velasco N, 1984 (N=91)	ROBS	1975-1982	Patients receiving cadaver renal transplants	RBT ≥5 (69) RBT<5 (31)‡	Concurrent	No	No	Poor
Cheigh JS, 1983 (N=62)	ROBS	1975-1982	Patients receiving cadaver renal transplant	RBT (24) NT (76)	Concurrent	No	No	Poor
Cho SI, 1983 (N=NR)	ROBS	1976-1981	Patients receiving primary cadaver renal transplants	RBT (NR) NT (NR)	Concurrent	No	No	Poor
Garvin PJ, 1983 (N=92)	ROBS	1977-1981	Patients receiving living-donor and cadaver renal transplants	RBT (77) NT (23)	Concurrent	No	No	Poor
Kerman RH, 1983 (N=104)	ROBS	NR	Patients receiving cadaver renal transplants	RBT >5 (49) RBT <5 (51)‡	Concurrent	No	No	Poor
Madsen M, 1983 (N=158)	POBS	1978-1982	Patients receiving cadaver renal transplants	RBT (90) NT (10)	Concurrent	No	No	Poor
Muller GA, 1983 (N=80)	ROBS	NR	Patients receiving cadaver renal transplants	RBT ≥4 (41) RBT 0-3 (59)‡	Concurrent	No	No	Poor
Myburgh JA, 1983 (N=262)	ROBS	1966-1982	Patients receiving cadaver renal transplants	RBT (74) NT (26)	Concurrent	No	Yes	Poor
Nubé MJ, 1983 (N=55)	POBS	1972-1981	Patients receiving primary cadaver renal transplants	LT (27) RBT (47) NT (25)	Historical	No	Yes	Poor
Okiye SE, 1983 (N=165)	ROBS	1968-1981	Patients receiving primary renal transplants	RBT (79) NT (21)	Concurrent	No	No	Poor
Rao KV, 1983 (N=300)	ROBS	1965-1980	Patients receiving renal transplants	NR	Concurrent	Yes	No	Poor

Study, Year (N=)	Study Design	Study Period	Population	Transfusion type* Exp (%) Control (%)	Type of control groups	Accounted for confounding	Demographic data in both groups†	Validity of the study
Richie RE, 1983 (N=452)	ROBS	1977-1981	Patients receiving cadaver or living-donor renal transplants	RBT (63) NT (37)	Concurrent	No	No	Poor
Spees EK, 1983 (N=2,406)	ROBS	1977-1982	Patients receiving cadaver renal transplants	RBT (80) NT (20)	Concurrent	No	No	Poor
Zeichner WD, 1983 (N=77)	ROBS	NR	Patients receiving primary cadaver renal transplants	RBT (79) NT (21)	Concurrent	No	No	Poor
Betuel H, 1982 (N=54)	ROBS	1977-1981	Patients receiving primary cadaver renal transplants	RBT (74) NT (26)	Concurrent	No	No	Poor
Chu D, 1982 (N=32)	POBS	1977-after	Patients receiving renal transplants	RBT (69) NT (31)	Concurrent	No	No	Poor
d'Apice 1982 (N=54)	ROBS	1977-1980	Dialysis patients who had not received transplants prior to study	PT (100)	Concurrent	No	No	Poor
Dewar PJ, 1982 (N=276)	ROBS	1969-1980	Patients receiving primary cadaver renal transplants	RBT (68) NT (32)	Concurrent	No	No	Poor
Fehrman I, 1982 (N=130)	ROBS	1970-1981	Patients receiving living-related renal transplants	RBT (65) NT (35)	Concurrent	No	No	Poor
Flechner SM, 1982 (N=384)	ROBS	1976-1979	Patients receiving primary cadaver renal transplants	RBT (66) NT (34)	Concurrent	No	No	Poor
Fradet Y, 1982 (N=121)	ROBS	1973-1980	Patients receiving primary cadaver renal transplants	RBT (77) NT (23)	Concurrent	No	Yes	Poor
Frisk B, 1982 (N=237)	ROBS	1977-1981	Patients receiving primary, 1-haplotype-matched cadaver renal transplants	PT (33) RBT (62) NT (5)	Concurrent	No	No	Poor
Fuller TC, 1982 (N=156)	ROBS	1976-1981	Patients receiving primary cadaver or HLA haploidentical living-related renal transplants	RBT (87) NT (13)	Historical	No	No	Poor

Study, Year (N=)	Study Design	Study Period	Population	Transfusion type* Exp (%) Control (%)	Type of control groups	Accounted for confounding	Demographic data in both groups†	Validity of the study
Glass NR, 1982 (N=94)	ROBS	1975-1980	Patients receiving primary cadaver renal transplants	RBT (48) NT (52)	Concurrent	No	Yes	Poor
Kovithavongs T, 1982 (N=28)	ROBS	NR	Patients receiving living-related, HLA haploidentical renal transplants	RBT (89) NT (11)	Concurrent	No	No	Poor
Mendez R, 1982 (N=67)	POBS	1978-1980	Patients receiving primary cadaver renal transplants	PT (28) RBT (36) PT + RBT (16) NT (19)	Concurrent	No	No	Poor
Sirchia G, 1982 (N=45)	POBS	1981-NR	Patients, treated with periodic hemodialysis, suffering from end-stage renal failure, on admission to the waiting list for primary cadaver renal transplant	PT (76) NT (24)	Historical	No	No	Poor
Takahashi I, 1982 (N=39)	POBS	1979-1981	Patients receiving 1-haplotype mismatched living donor renal transplants	DST (59) NT (41)	Concurrent	Yes	No	Poor
Walker JF, 1982 (N=204)	ROBS	1969-1979	Patients receiving HD or PD prior to receiving cadaver renal transplants	RBT (67) NT (33)	Concurrent	No	No	Poor
Feduska, 1981 (N= 732)	ROBS	1970-1980	Patients receiving primary cadaveric renal transplants	RBT (71) NT (29)	Concurrent	No	No	Poor
Hurst PE, 1981 (N=168)	ROBS	1967-1978	Patients receiving cadaver renal transplants	RBT (65) NT (35)	Concurrent	No	Yes	Poor
Persijn GG, 1981 (N=52)	POBS	1977-NR	Patients receiving cadaver renal transplants	LT (77) LF (23)	Concurrent	No	Yes	Fair
Sirchia G, 1981 (N=484)	ROBS	1972-1977	Patients receiving cadaver renal transplants	RBT (67) NT (33)	Concurrent	No	No	Poor

Study, Year (N=)	Study Design	Study Period	Population	Transfusion type* Exp (%) Control (%)	Type of control groups	Accounted for confounding	Demographic data in both groups†	Validity of the study
Thorsby E, 1981 (N=129)	ROBS	NR	Patients receiving primary cadaver renal transplants	RBT (57) NT (43)	Concurrent	No	No	Poor
Van Es A, 1981 (N=124)	ROBS	1966-1980	Patients receiving primary cadaver renal transplants	RBT (80) NT (20)	Concurrent	No	No	Poor
Corry RJ, 1980 (N=94)	ROBS	1973-1980	Patients receiving primary cadaver renal transplants	RBT (45) NT (49)	Concurrent	No	No	Poor
Fehman I, 1980 (N=229)	ROBS	1970-1978	Patients receiving primary cadaver renal transplants	RBT (69) NT (31)	Concurrent	No	Yes	Poor
Jakobsen A, 1980 (N=301)	ROBS	1965-1977	Renal transplant recipients with polycystic renal diseases	RBT (52) NT (48)	Concurrent	No	No	Poor
Salvatierra O, 1980 (N=57)	ROBS	NR	Patients receiving one-haplotype matched living-related donor renal transplants	DST (40) NT (60)	Concurrent	No	Yes	Poor
Solheim BG, 1980 (N=191)	ROBS	1969-1977	Patients receiving primary living-related renal transplants	RBT (45) NT (55)	Concurrent	No	Yes	Poor
Solheim BG, 1980 (N=348)	ROBS	1969-1978	Patients receiving primary cadaver renal transplants	RBT (47) NT (53)	Concurrent	No	Yes	Poor
Spees EK, 1980 (N=995)	ROBS	1977-1979	Patients receiving cadaver renal transplants	RBT (83) NT (17)	Concurrent	No	Yes	Poor
Andrus C, 1979 (N=55)	ROBS	1971-1974	Patients receiving well-matched cadaver renal transplants	RBT > 5 (73) RBT < 5 (27)‡	Concurrent	No	No	Poor
Fauchet R, 1979 (N=66)	ROBS	1972-1977	Patients receiving renal transplants	RBT (61) NT (39)	Concurrent	No	Yes	Poor

C - 11

Study, Year (N=)	Study Design	Study Period	Population	Transfusion type* Exp (%) Control (%)	Type of control groups	Accounted for confounding	Demographic data in both groups†	Validity of the study
Houmant M, 1979 (N=163)	ROBS	NR	Patients receiving cadaver renal transplants	RBT (74) NT (26)	Concurrent	No	No	Poor
Oei LS, 1979 ‖ (N=86)	ROBS	1973-1979	Patients receiving living-related renal transplants	RBT (80) NT (20)	Concurrent	No	No	Poor
Sengar D, 1979 (N=117)	ROBS	1969-NR	Patients receiving primary cadaver renal transplant	RBT (67) NT (33)	Concurrent	No	No	Poor
Werner-Favre C, 1979 (N=101)	POBS	1976-1978	Patients receiving primary cadaver renal transplants	RBT (86) NT (14)	Concurrent	No	No	Poor
Blamey RW, 1978 (N=32)	ROBS	1974-1977	Patients receiving primary cadaver renal transplants	RBT (31) NT (69)	Concurrent	No	No	Poor
Briggs JD, 1978 (N=83)	ROBS	1969-1975	Patients receiving cadaver renal transplants	RBT (82) NT (18)	Concurrent	No	No	Poor
Jeffery JR, 1978 (N=48)	ROBS	1975-1977	Patients receiving primary cadaver renal transplant	RBT (50) NT (50)	Concurrent	No	Yes	Poor
Jeffrey JR, 1978 (N=44)	ROBS	NR	Patients receiving primary cadaver renal transplant	RBT (45) NT (55)	Concurrent	No	No	Poor
Stiller CR, 1978 (N=32)	ROBS	NR	Patients receiving cadaver renal transplants	RBT (44) NT (56)	Concurrent	No	No	Poor
Brynger H, 1977 (N=244)	ROBS	1966-1976	Patients receiving primary renal transplants	RBT (76) NT (24)	Concurrent	No	Yes	Poor
Fuller TC, 1977 (N=90)	ROBS	1969-1975	Patients receiving primary cadaver renal transplants	RBT (89) NT (11)	Concurrent	No	No	Poor

Study, Year (N=)	Study Design	Study Period	Population	Transfusion type* Exp (%) Control (%)	Type of control groups	Accounted for confounding	Demographic data in both groups[†]	Validity of the study
Husberg BO, 1977 (N=95)	ROBS	1968-1976	Non-diabetic patients receiving primary cadaver renal transplants	RBT (68) NT (32)	Historical	No	No	Poor
Joysey VC, 1977 (N=272)	ROBS	1965-1976	Patients receiving primary cadaver renal transplants	RBT (60) NT (40)	Concurrent	No	No	Poor
Perkins HA, 1977 (N=126)	ROBS	NR	Patients on chronic dialysis, receiving primary renal transplant	RBT (79) NT (21)	Concurrent	No	No	Poor
Persijn GG, 1977 (N=622)	ROBS	1967-1975	Patients receiving primary cadaver renal transplant	RBT (95) NT (5)	Concurrent	No	Yes	Poor
Polesky HF, 1977 (N=77)	ROBS	1973-1976	Patients receiving primary renal transplant	RBT (52) LT (17) NT (31)	Concurrent	No	No	Poor
Sachs JA, 1977 (N=524)	POBS	1969-1976	Patients receiving HLA-matched cadaver renal transplants	RBT (68) NT (32)	Concurrent	No	No	Poor
Säfwenberg J, 1977 (N=115)	ROBS	NR	Patients receiving primary cadaver renal transplant	RBT (55) NT (45)	Concurrent	No	No	Poor
Walter S, 1977 (N=88)	ROBS	1970-1976	Patients receiving primary cadaver renal transplant	RBT (74) NT (26)	Concurrent	No	No	Poor
Opelz G, 1974 (N=290)	ROBS	1970-1974	Patients receiving primary cadaver renal transplant	RBT (79) NT (21)	Concurrent	No	No	Poor
Opelz G, 1973 (N=148)	ROBS	1969-1971	Patients receiving cadaver renal transplants	RBT (83) NT (17)	Concurrent	No	No	Poor
Oplez G, 1973 (N=144)	ROBS	NR	Patients receiving cadaveric renal transplants	NR	NR	No	No	Poor
Opelz, 1972 (N=829)	ROBS	NR	Patients receiving primary cadaveric renal transplants	NR	NR	No	No	Poor

* Transfusion data included experimental group(s) versus control group used in the analyses of this report
[†] Demographic data in relation to the transfusion populations.
[‡] Different number/units of transfusions were evaluated in the analyses

C - 13

§ The validity of the study was graded as fair quality due to the extended followup time period (10 years) and included a large population from the UCLA transplant registry.
‖Repeated transfusion group versus control group
¶Analysis only reported results of living-related donor renal transplants, results of cadaveric donor transplants were not evaluated due to overlapping population with Corry RJ et al. 1980.

ADPKD=autosomal dominant polycystic kidney disease, CCT=clinical controlled trial, CyA=cyclosporine, DST=donor specific transfusion, ESRD=end stage renal disease, HD=hemodialysis, HLA=human leukocyte antigen, LT=leukocyte-depleted transfusion, LF=leukocyte-free transfusion, MMF=mycophenolatemofetil, MV=multivariate analysis, N=total number of patients included in the analyses of the study, NR=not reported, NT=no transfusion, PD=peritoneal dialysis, POBS=prospective observational study, PT=protocol transfusion, RBT= random blood transfusion, ROBS=retrospective observational study, SLE=systemic lupus erythematosus, Tac=tacrolimus.

Appendix D. Strength of Evidence Tables

Appendix Table 1. Strength of evidence for the impact of transfusion (any kinds) on renal allograft outcomes in kidney (with or without pancreas) transplant recipients (KQ1a)

Outcome	Number of Analyses	Study Design	Quality			Assessment		Summary of Findings
			Risk of Bias	Consistency		Directness	Precision	Quality
Significant impact on any rejection	25	4 CCT 1 POBS 16 ROBS	Serious limitation	Very serious inconsistency		No indirectness	NA	Low
Direction of impact on any rejection*	47	8 CCT 1 POBS 26 ROBS	Serious limitation	Very serious inconsistency		No indirectness	NA	Insufficient
Significant impact on 1-year graft survival	55	4 CCT 6 POBS 38 ROBS	Serious limitation	Very serious inconsistency		No indirectness	NA	Low
Magnitude of impact on 1-year graft survival	132	9 CCT 9 POBS 72 ROBS	Serious limitation	Very serious inconsistency		No indirectness	NA	Low
Significant impact on max duration graft survival	65	4 CCT 6 POBS 44 ROBS	Serious limitation	Very serious inconsistency		No indirectness	NA	Low
Magnitude of impact on max duration graft survival	146	10 CCT 11 POBS 80 ROBS	Serious limitation	Very serious inconsistency		No indirectness	NA	Low
Significant impact on 1-year patient survival	16	2 CCT 1 POBS 10 ROBS	Serious limitation	Very serious inconsistency		No indirectness	NA	Low
Magnitude of impact on 1-year patient survival	35	7 CCT 1 POBS 19 ROBS	Serious limitation	Very serious inconsistency		No indirectness	NA	Low

Outcome	Number of Analyses	Study Design	Quality				Summary of Findings
			Risk of Bias	Consistency	Assessment Directness	Precision	Quality
Significant impact on max duration patient survival	18	1 CCT 2 POBS 13 ROBS	Serious limitation	Very serious inconsistency	No indirectness	NA	Low
Magnitude of impact on max duration patient survival	41	7 CCT 2 POBS 23 ROBS	Serious limitation	Very serious inconsistency	No indirectness	NA	Low

*Insufficient data since it was difficult to gauge the magnitude of the effect from the available data
CCT=clinical controlled trials, NA=not applicable, POBS=prospective observational studies, ROBS=retrospective observational studies

Appendix Table 2. Strength of evidence for the impact of therapeutic transfusion (excluding donor-specific transfusion analyses) on renal allograft outcomes (KQ1a)

Outcome	Number of Analyses	Study Design	Quality				Summary of Findings
			Risk of Bias	Consistency	Assessment Directness	Precision	Quality
Significant impact on any rejection	14	1 CCT 0 POBS 12 ROBS	Serious limitation	Very serious inconsistency	No indirectness	NA	Low
Direction of impact on any rejection*	20	3 CCT 0 POBS 14 ROBS	Serious limitation	Very serious inconsistency	No indirectness	NA	Insufficient
Significant impact on 1-year graft survival	43	3 CCT 4 POBS 32 ROBS	Serious limitation	Very serious inconsistency	No indirectness	NA	Low
Magnitude of impact on 1-year graft survival	99	5 CCT 7 POBS 60 ROBS	Serious limitation	Very serious inconsistency	No indirectness	NA	Low
Significant impact on max duration graft survival	47	3 CCT 4 POBS 34 ROBS	Serious limitation	Very serious inconsistency	No indirectness	NA	Low

Outcome	Number of Analyses	Study Design	Quality			Assessment		Summary of Findings
			Risk of Bias	Consistency	Directness	Precision		Quality
Magnitude of impact on **max duration graft survival**	105	5 CCT 9 POBS 63 ROBS	Serious limitation	Very serious inconsistency	No indirectness	NA		Low
Significant impact on **1-year patient survival**	12	1 CCT 0 POBS 9 ROBS	Serious limitation	Very serious inconsistency	No indirectness	NA		Low
Magnitude of impact on **1-year patient survival**	20	2 CCT 0 POBS 13 ROBS	Serious limitation	Very serious inconsistency	No indirectness	NA		Low
Significant impact on **max duration patient survival**	12	0 CCT 0 POBS 11 ROBS	Serious limitation	Very serious inconsistency	No indirectness	NA		Low
Magnitude of impact on **max duration patient survival**	23	2 CCT 1 POBS 14 ROBS	Serious limitation	Very serious inconsistency	No indirectness	NA		Low

*Insufficient data since it was difficult to gauge the magnitude of the effect from the available data
CCT=clinical controlled trials, NA=not applicable, POBS=prospective observational studies, ROBS=retrospective observational studies

Appendix Table 3. Strength of evidence for the impact of donor-specific transfusion versus therapeutic transfusion on renal allograft outcomes in kidney transplant recipients (KQ 1bi)

Outcome	Number of Analyses	Study Design	Quality Assessment				Summary of Findings
			Risk of Bias	Consistency	Directness	Precision	Quality
Significant impact on **any rejection**	3	0 CCT 0 POBS 3 ROBS	Serious limitation	Serious inconsistency	No indirectness	NA	Low
Direction of impact on **any rejection***	7	0 CCT 0 POBS 6 ROBS	Serious limitation	Very serious inconsistency	No indirectness	NA	Insufficient
Significant impact on **1-year graft survival**	4	0 CCT 0 POBS 4 ROBS	Serious limitation	Serious inconsistency	No indirectness	NA	Low
Magnitude of impact on **1-year graft survival**	16	0 CCT 1 POBS 9 ROBS	Serious limitation	Very serious inconsistency	No indirectness	NA	Low
Significant impact on **max duration graft survival**	5	0 CCT 0 POBS 5 ROBS	Serious limitation	Very serious inconsistency	No indirectness	NA	Low
Magnitude of impact on **max duration graft survival**	17	0 CCT 1 POBS 10 ROBS	Serious limitation	Very serious inconsistency	No indirectness	NA	Low
Significant impact on **1-year patient survival**	2	0 CCT 0 POBS 2 ROBS	Serious limitation	Serious inconsistency	No indirectness	NA	Insufficient
Magnitude of impact on **1-year patient survival**	4	0 CCT 0 POBS 3 ROBS	Serious limitation	Serious inconsistency	No indirectness	NA	Low
Significant impact on **max duration patient survival**	2	0 CCT 0 POBS 2 ROBS	Serious limitation	Serious inconsistency	No indirectness	NA	Insufficient

| Outcome | Number of Analyses | Study Design | Quality | | | | Summary of Findings |
			Risk of Bias	Consistency	Directness	Precision	Quality
Magnitude of impact on max duration patient survival	4	0 CCT 0 POBS 3 ROBS	Serious limitation	Serious inconsistency	No indirectness	NA	Low

*Insufficient data since it was difficult to gauge the magnitude of the effect from the available data
CCT=clinical controlled trials, NA=not applicable, POBS=prospective observational studies, ROBS=retrospective observational studies

Appendix Table 4. Strength of evidence for the impact of number of transfusion on renal allograft outcomes in kidney transplant recipients (KQ 1bii)

| Outcome | Number of Analyses | Study Design | Quality | | | | Summary of Findings |
			Risk of Bias	Consistency	Directness	Precision	Quality
Any versus Any number of transfusion							
Significant impact on any rejection	5	0 CCT 0 POBS 2 ROBS	Serious limitation	Very Serious inconsistency	No indirectness	NA	Low
Direction of impact on any rejection*	18	0 CCT 0 POBS 4 ROBS	Very Serious limitation	Very serious inconsistency	No indirectness	NA	Insufficient
Any number vs. no transfusion							
Significant impact on 1-year graft survival	12	0 CCT 0 POBS 6 ROBS	Serious limitation	Very serious inconsistency	No indirectness	NA	Low
Magnitude of impact on 1-year graft survival	51	1 CCT 1 POBS 16 ROBS	Serious limitation	Very serious inconsistency	No indirectness	NA	Low
Significant impact on max duration graft survival	9	0 CCT 0 POBS 6 ROBS	Serious limitation	Very serious inconsistency	No indirectness	NA	Low

Outcome	Number of Analyses	Study Design	Quality			Precision	Summary of Findings Quality
			Risk of Bias	Consistency	Directness		
Magnitude of impact on **max duration graft survival**	53	1 CCT 1 POBS 17 ROBS	Serious limitation	Very serious inconsistency	No indirectness	NA	Low
Significant impact on **1-year patient survival**	8	0 CCT 0 POBS 3 ROBS	Serious limitation	Very serious inconsistency	No indirectness	NA	Low
Magnitude of impact on **1-year patient survival**	8	0 CCT 0 POBS 3 ROBS	Serious limitation	Very serious inconsistency	No indirectness	NA	Low
Significant impact on **max duration patient survival**	8	0 CCT 0 POBS 3 ROBS	Serious limitation	Very serious inconsistency	No indirectness	NA	Low
Magnitude of impact on **max duration patient survival**	7	0 CCT 0 POBS 3 ROBS	Serious limitation	Very serious inconsistency	No indirectness	NA	Low
Higher versus lower transfusion intensity							
Significant impact on **1-year graft survival**	11	0 CCT 0 POBS 6 ROBS	Serious limitation	Very serious inconsistency	No indirectness	NA	Low
Magnitude of impact on **1-year graft survival**	43	1 CCT 1 POBS 18 ROBS	Serious limitation	Very serious inconsistency	No indirectness	NA	Low
Significant impact on **max duration graft survival**	9	1 CCT 0 POBS 6 ROBS	Serious limitation	Very serious inconsistency	No indirectness	NA	Low
Magnitude of impact on **max duration graft survival**	47	2 CCT 1 POBS 21 ROBS	Serious limitation	Very serious inconsistency	No indirectness	NA	Low
Significant impact on **1-year patient survival**	7	0 CCT 0 POBS 3 ROBS	Serious limitation	Very serious inconsistency	No indirectness	NA	Low

Outcome	Number of Analyses	Study Design	Quality				Summary of Findings
			Risk of Bias	Consistency	Assessment Directness	Precision	Quality
Magnitude of impact on **1-year patient survival**	7	0 CCT 0 POBS 3 ROBS	Serious limitation	Very serious inconsistency	No indirectness	NA	Low
Significant impact on **max duration patient survival**	7	0 CCT 0 POBS 3 ROBS	Serious limitation	Very serious inconsistency	No indirectness	NA	Low
Magnitude of impact on **max duration patient survival**	5	0 CCT 0 POBS 3 ROBS	Serious limitation	Very serious inconsistency	No indirectness	NA	Low

*Insufficient data since it was difficult to gauge the magnitude of the effect from the available data
CCT=clinical controlled trials, NA=not applicable, POBS=prospective observational studies, ROBS=retrospective observational studies

Appendix Table 5. Strength of evidence for the impact of unit of transfusion on renal allograft outcomes in kidney transplant recipients (KQ 1bii)

Outcome	Number of Analyses	Study Design	Quality				Summary of Findings
			Risk of Bias	Consistency	Assessment Directness	Precision	Quality
Any versus any transfusion units							
Significant impact on **any rejection**	1	1 CCT 0 POBS 0 ROBS	Very serious limitation	NA	No indirectness	NA	Insufficient
Direction of impact on **any rejection***	1	1 CCT 0 POBS 0 ROBS	Very serious limitation	NA	No indirectness	NA	Insufficient
Any units versus no transfusion							
Significant impact on **1-year graft survival**	11	0 CCT 0 POBS 4 ROBS	Serious limitation	Very serious inconsistency	No indirectness	NA	Low

Outcome	Number of Analyses	Study Design	Quality				Summary of Findings
			Risk of Bias	Consistency	Directness	Precision	Quality
Magnitude of impact on **1-year graft survival**	21	1 CCT 0 POBS 8 ROBS	Serious limitation	Very serious inconsistency	No indirectness	NA	Low
Significant impact on **max duration graft survival**	16	1 CCT 0 POBS 6 ROBS	Serious limitation	Very serious inconsistency	No indirectness	NA	Low
Magnitude of impact on **max duration graft survival**	22	1 CCT 1 POBS 8 ROBS	Serious limitation	Very serious inconsistency	No indirectness	NA	Low
Significant impact on **1-year patient survival**	0	---	---	---	---	---	Insufficient
Magnitude of impact on **1-year patient survival**	0	---	---	---	---	---	Insufficient
Significant impact on **max duration patient survival**	0	---	---	---	---	---	Insufficient
Magnitude of impact on **max duration patient survival**	0	---	---	---	---	---	Insufficient
Higher versus lower transfusion units							
Significant impact on **1-year graft survival**	6	0 CCT 0 POBS 3 ROBS	Serious limitation	Very serious inconsistency	No indirectness	NA	Low
Magnitude of impact on **1-year graft survival**	12	1 CCT 0 POBS 7 ROBS	Serious limitation	Very serious inconsistency	No indirectness	NA	Low
Significant impact on **max duration graft survival**	12	1 CCT 0 POBS 5 ROBS	Serious limitation	Very serious inconsistency	No indirectness	NA	Low

Outcome	Number of Analyses	Study Design	Quality			Assessment		Summary of Findings
			Risk of Bias	Consistency	Directness	Precision		Quality
Magnitude of impact on **max duration graft survival**	16	1 CCT 0 POBS 9 ROBS	Serious limitation	Very serious inconsistency	No indirectness	NA		Low
Significant impact on **1-year patient survival**	0	---	---	---	---	---		Insufficient
Magnitude of impact on **1-year patient survival**	0	---	---	---	---	---		Insufficient
Significant impact on **max duration patient survival**	0	---	---	---	---	---		Insufficient
Magnitude of impact on **max duration patient survival**	0	---	---	---	---	---		Insufficient

*Insufficient data since it was difficult to gauge the magnitude of the effect from the available data
CCT=clinical controlled trials, NA=not applicable, POBS=prospective observational studies, ROBS=retrospective observational studies

Appendix Table 6. Strength of evidence for the impact of number of donors on renal allograft outcomes in kidney transplant recipients (KQ 1bii)

Outcome	Number of Analyses	Study Design	Quality			Assessment		Summary of Findings
			Risk of Bias	Consistency	Directness	Precision		Quality
Significant impact on **any rejection**	0	---	---	---	---	---		Insufficient
Direction of impact on **any rejection**	0	---	---	---	---	---		Insufficient
Significant impact on **1-year graft survival**	0	---	---	---	---	---		Insufficient
Magnitude of impact on **1-year graft survival**	0	---	---	---	---	---		Insufficient

Appendix Table 7. Strength of evidence for the impact of leukocyte-depleted transfusion on renal allograft outcomes in kidney transplant recipients (KQ 1biii)

Outcome	Number of Analyses	Study Design	Risk of Bias	Quality Assessment Consistency	Directness	Precision	Summary of Findings Quality
Significant impact on **max duration graft survival**	0	---	---	---	---	---	Insufficient
Magnitude of impact on **max duration graft survival**	0	---	---	---	---	---	Insufficient
Significant impact on **1-year patient survival**	0	---	---	---	---	---	Insufficient
Magnitude of impact on **1-year patient survival**	0	---	---	---	---	---	Insufficient
Significant impact on **max duration patient survival**	0	---	---	---	---	---	Insufficient
Magnitude of impact on **max duration patient survival**	0	---	---	---	---	---	Insufficient

Leukocyte depleted blood versus no transfusions

Outcome	Number of Analyses	Study Design	Risk of Bias	Quality Assessment Consistency	Directness	Precision	Summary of Findings Quality
Significant impact on **any rejection**	0	---	---	---	---	---	Insufficient
Direction of impact on **any rejection**	0	---	---	---	---	---	Insufficient
Significant impact on **1-year graft survival**	0	---	---	---	---	---	Insufficient

Outcome	Number of Analyses	Study Design	Quality		Assessment		Summary of Findings
			Risk of Bias	Consistency	Directness	Precision	Quality
Magnitude of impact on **1-year graft survival**	2	0 CCT 1 POBS 1 ROBS	Serious limitation	Serious inconsistency	No indirectness	NA	Low
Significant impact on **max duration graft survival**	0	---	---	---	---	---	Insufficient
Magnitude of impact on **max duration graft survival**	2	0 CCT 1 POBS 1 ROBS	Serious limitation	Serious inconsistency	No indirectness	NA	Low
Significant impact on **1-year patient survival**	0	---	---	---	---	---	Insufficient
Magnitude of impact on **1-year patient survival**	0	---	---	---	---	---	Insufficient
Significant impact on **max duration patient survival**	1	0 CCT 1 POBS 0 ROBS	Serious limitation	NA	No indirectness	NA	Insufficient
Magnitude of impact on **max duration patient survival**	1	0 CCT 1 POBS 0 ROBS	Serious limitation	NA	No indirectness	NA	Insufficient
Leukocyte depleted versus therapeutic transfusions							
Significant impact on **any rejection**	0	---	---	---	---	---	Insufficient
Direction of impact on **any rejection**	0	---	---	---	---	---	Insufficient
Significant impact on **1-year graft survival**	1	0 CCT 1 POBS 0 ROBS	Serious limitation	NA	No indirectness	NA	Insufficient
Magnitude of impact on **1-year graft survival**	2	0 CCT 1 POBS 1 ROBS	Serious limitation	Serious inconsistency	No indirectness	NA	Low

| Outcome | Number of Analyses | Study Design | Quality | | | | Summary of Findings |
			Risk of Bias	Consistency	Assessment Directness	Precision	Quality
Significant impact on **max duration graft survival**	1	0 CCT 1 POBS 0 ROBS	Serious limitation	NA	No indirectness	NA	Insufficient
Magnitude of impact on **max duration graft survival**	2	0 CCT 1 POBS 1 ROBS	Serious limitation	Serious inconsistency	No indirectness	NA	Low
Significant impact on **1-year patient survival**	0	---	---	---	---	---	Insufficient
Magnitude of impact on **1-year patient survival**	0	---	---	---	---	---	Insufficient
Significant impact on **max duration patient survival**	1	0 CCT 1 POBS 0 ROBS	Serious limitation	NA	No indirectness	NA	Insufficient
Magnitude of impact on **max duration patient survival**	1	0 CCT 1 POBS 0 ROBS	Serious limitation	NA	No indirectness	NA	Insufficient

CCT=clinical controlled trials, LDT=leukocyte depleted transfusion, NA=not applicable, POBS=prospective observational studies, ROBS=retrospective observational studies, Txn=transfusion

Appendix Table 8. Strength of evidence for the impact of transfusion over different time periods on renal allograft outcomes in kidney transplant recipients (KQ 1biv-v)

| Outcome | Number of Analyses | Study Design | Quality | | | | Summary of Findings |
			Risk of Bias	Consistency	Assessment Directness	Precision	Quality
Significant impact on **any rejection**	11	1 CCT 0 POBS 8 ROBS	Serious limitation	Very serious inconsistency	No indirectness	NA	Low
Direction of impact on **any rejection***	35	7 CCT 0 POBS 20 ROBS	Serious limitation	Very serious inconsistency	No indirectness	NA	Low

			Quality		Assessment		Summary of Findings
Outcome	Number of Analyses	Study Design	Risk of Bias	Consistency	Directness	Precision	Quality
Significant impact on **1-year graft survival**	47	3 CCT 5 POBS 34 ROBS	Serious limitation	Very serious inconsistency	No indirectness	NA	Low
Magnitude of impact on **1-year graft survival**	108	8 CCT 7 POBS 66 ROBS	Serious limitation	Very serious inconsistency	No indirectness	NA	Low
Significant impact on **max duration graft survival**	57	3 CCT 5 POBS 40 ROBS	Serious limitation	Very serious inconsistency	No indirectness	NA	Low
Magnitude of impact on **max duration graft survival**	119	8 CCT 9 POBS 73 ROBS	Serious limitation	Very serious inconsistency	No indirectness	NA	Low
Significant impact on **1-year patient survival**	17	2 CCT 1 POBS 10 ROBS	Serious limitation	Very serious inconsistency	No indirectness	NA	Low
Magnitude of impact on **1-year patient survival**	30	6 CCT 1 POBS 17 ROBS	Serious limitation	Very serious inconsistency	No indirectness	NA	Low
Significant impact on **max duration patient survival**	18	1 CCT 1 POBS 14 ROBS	Serious limitation	Very serious inconsistency	No indirectness	NA	Low
Magnitude of impact on **max duration patient survival**	37	6 CCT 2 POBS 22 ROBS	Serious limitation	Very serious inconsistency	No indirectness	NA	Low

*Insufficient data since it was difficult to gauge the magnitude of the effect from the available data
CCT=clinical controlled trials, NA=not applicable, POBS=prospective observational studies, ROBS=retrospective observational studies

Appendix Table 9. Strength of evidence for the impact of PRA assays in predicting renal allograft outcomes in kidney (with or without pancreas) transplant recipients (KQ2b)

Outcome	Number of Analyses	Study Design	Quality Risk of Bias	Consistency	Assessment Directness	Precision	Summary of Findings Quality
Significant impact on **1-year** rejection	1	1 CCT	Serious limitation	NA	No indirectness	NA	Low
Significant impact on **max duration** rejection	2	1 CCT 1 ROBS	Serious limitation	Very serious inconsistency	No indirectness	NA	Low
Direction of impact on **1-year rejection***	1	1 CCT	Serious limitation	NA	No indirectness	NA	Insufficient
Direction of impact on **max duration rejection***	2	1 CCT 1 ROBS	Serious limitation	Very serious inconsistency	No indirectness	NA	Insufficient
Significant impact on **1-year** graft survival	5	1 CCT 3 ROBS	Serious limitation	Very serious inconsistency	No indirectness	NA	Low
Significant impact on **max duration** graft survival	9	1 CCT 6 ROBS	Serious limitation	Very serious inconsistency	No indirectness	NA	Low
Direction of impact on **1-year** graft survival	8	1 CCT 6 ROBS	Serious limitation	Very serious inconsistency	No indirectness	NA	Low
Direction of impact on **max duration** graft survival	14	1 CCT 10 ROBS	Serious limitation	Very serious inconsistency	No indirectness	NA	Low
Significant impact on **1-year** patient Survival	2	1 ROBS	Serious limitation	NA	No indirectness	NA	Low

Outcome	Number of Analyses	Study Design	Quality		Assessment		Summary of Findings
			Risk of Bias	Consistency	Directness	Precision	Quality
Significant impact on Max duration patient survival	2	1 ROBS	Serious limitation	NA	No indirectness	NA	Low
Direction of impact on 1-year patient survival	2	1 ROBS	Serious limitation	NA	No indirectness	NA	Low
Magnitude of impact on max duration patient survival	2	1 ROBS	Serious limitation	NA	No indirectness	NA	Low

*Insufficient data since it was difficult to gauge the magnitude of the effect from the available data
CCT=clinical controlled trials, NA=not applicable, PRA = Panel Reactive Antibodies, ROBS=retrospective observational studies

Appendix E. Sensitization Tables

Other results depicting the impact of sensitization on eligibility for transplantation in transfused patients

Study, Year (N=)	Type of transfusion	Number of transfused patients ($N_T=$)	Assessment	Number of transfused patients who were sensitized N_S/N_T (%)	Number of sensitized patients who were transplanted with planned kidney n/Ns (%)	Number of sensitized patients who were not transplanted with planned kidney n/Ns (%)	Comments
Eisenberger U, 2009 (N=138)	DST	69	PRA >0%	4/69 (5.8)	4/4 (100)	0/4 (0)	All patients included in the study were transplanted
Tang H, 2008 (N=2,882)	NR	NR	Peak PRA level	NR	NR	NR	NA
Waanders MM, 2008 (N=118)	HLA-DR matched transfusion	49	PRA: highest and most recent	NR	NR	NR	NA
El-Husseini AA, 2005 (N=282)	RT	166	Lymphocytotoxic crossmatch	NR	NR	NR	Patients with positive lymphocytotoxic crossmatches were considered as sensitized, and thus excluded from the study
Opelz G, 2005 (N= 164,534)	RT	NR	Preformed antibodies defined as PRA 1-50% or > 50%	NR	NR	NR	NA
Higgins RM, 2004 (N=265)	RT	NR	NR	NR	NR	NR	NA
Park YH, 2004 (N=77)	RT	14	NR	NR	NR	NR	NA
Bunnapradist S, 2003 (N=7,079)	RT	NR	PRA 0-10 PRA 11-30 PRA > 30%	NR	NR	NR	NA

Study, Year (N=)	Type of transfusion	Number of transfused patients (N_T=)	Assessment	Number of transfused patients who were sensitized N_s/N_T (%)	Number of sensitized patients who were transplanted with planned kidney n/Ns (%)	Number of sensitized patients who were not transplanted with planned kidney n/Ns (%)	Comments
Herget-Rosenthal S, 2003 (N=40)	RT	NR	NR	NR	NR	NR	NA
Lietz K, 2003 (N=502)	RT	NR	PRA - maximum, minimum, and reactivity at the time of transplantation	NR	NR	NR	NA
Agarwal SK, 2002 (N=144)	RT	NR	NR	NR	NR	NR	NA
Barbari A, 2001 (N=84)	DST	64	Crossmatch	NR	NR	NR	NA
Hiesse C, 2001 (N=144)	HLA-DR matched or mismatched transfusion	97	Lymphocytotoxic anti-HLA antibodies (IgG anti-T cells)	1/70 (1.0)*	1/1 (100)	0/1 (0)	Cytotoxicity not reported in 27 patients, who were not transplanted at the end of study period
Poli L, 2001 (N=514)	RT	223	Crossmatch and PRA	NR	NR	NR	PRA and Crossmatch were both negative at the time of transplant
Montagnino G, 2000 (N=143)	RT	NR	PRA >50%	NR	NR	NR	NA
Alexander JW, 1999 (N=212)	DST	115	Peak PRA; positive T-cell crossmatch	NR	NR	NR	NA
de Mattos AM, 1999 (N=108)	RT	84	Peak PRA> 2%; crossmatch	NR	NR	NR	NA
Padányi A, 1998 (N=57)	DST	13	Anti-HLA cytotoxic antibody	NR	NR	NR	NA

E - 2

Study, Year (N=)	Type of transfusion	Number of transfused patients ($N_T=$)	Assessment	Number of transfused patients who were sensitized N_s/N_T (%)	Number of sensitized patients who were transplanted with planned kidney n/Ns (%)	Number of sensitized patients who were not transplanted with planned kidney n/Ns (%)	Comments
Chavers BM, 1997 (N=4015)	RT	2844	NR	NR	NR	NR	NA
Galvao M, 1997 (N=60)	DST	37	PRA and crossmatch	NR	NR	NR	NA
Opelz G, 1997 (N=654)	RT	321	Lymphocytotoxic antibodies: >11 % of test panel	13/205 (6.3)*	13/13 (100)	0/13 (0)	162 patients still waiting at the end of study period, 10 (6%) of them (transfusion status unknown) had PRA >10%
Sharma RK, 1997 (N=30)	DST	15	Lymphocytotoxic crossmatch against T, B, and T+B cells before transplant, before DST, 7 days & 4 weeks post-transplant	1/15 (6.7)	1/1 (100)	0/1 (0)	All patients included in the study were transplanted
Inoue S, 1996 (N=115)	DST	43	Crossmatches with the direct donor's B and T lymphocytes	NR	NR	NR	Patients were transplanted if crossmatch remained negative throughout the DST sessions.
Jin DC, 1996 (N=680)	DST	152	Cytotoxicity test	NR	NR	NR	NA
Peters TG, 1995 (N=17,937)	RT	NR	PRA >60%	NR	NR	NR	NA
Poli F, 1995 (N=416)	RT	204	PRA >0%	NR	NR	NR	NA
Barber WH, 1994 (N=598)	DST	288	NR	NR	NR	NR	NA
Kahn D, 1994 (N=52)	DST	33	Crossmatch	NR	NR	NR	NA

Study, Year (N=)	Type of transfusion	Number of transfused patients (N_T=)	Assessment	Number of transfused patients who were sensitized N_S/N_T (%)	Number of sensitized patients who were transplanted with planned kidney n/Ns (%)	Number of sensitized patients who were not transplanted with planned kidney n/Ns (%)	Comments
Sautner T, 1994 (N=146)	RT	NR	PRA 0 PRA 1-40 PRA > 40	NR	NR	NR	NA
Egidi MF, 1993 (N=284)	RT	236	NR	NR	NR	NR	NA
Basri N, 1992 (N=53)	DST	28	Crossmatch	NR	NR	NR	NA
Vathsala A, 1992 (N=116)	RT	NR	PRA > 60%; crossmatch	NR	NR	NR	NA
Velidedeoglu E, 1992 (N=437)	DST	344	Formation of antibodies against donor lymphocytes; crossmatch	NR	NR	NR	Patients were not transplanted with a positive crossmatch
Xiao X, 1992 (N=201)	RT	152	Lymphocytotoxic crossmatch	NR	NR	NR	NA
Garcia LF, 1991 (N=NR)	DST DST+RT RT	28 51 RT	Crossmatch	4/28 (14.3) 23/51 (45.1) NR	NR	NR	NA
Kerman RH, 1991 (N=365)	RT	242	Crossmatch; PRA against panel of 60	0/242 (0)	NA	NA	Retrospective study included all transplant recipients who had negative crossmatch
Sanfilippo F, 1990 (N=2138)	DST RT	430 315	PRA ≥ 60%	NR	NR	NR	NA
Kasai I, 1989 (N=26)	DST†	19	Crossmatch	NR	NR	NR	NA
Pfaff WW, 1989 a‡	PT	373	PRA 11-99%	33/373 (8.8)	NR	NR	NA

Study, Year (N=)	Type of transfusion	Number of transfused patients ($N_T=$)	Assessment	Number of transfused patients who were sensitized N_S/N_T (%)	Number of sensitized patients who were transplanted with planned kidney n/Ns (%)	Number of sensitized patients who were not transplanted with planned kidney n/Ns (%)	Comments
Pfaff WW, 1989 b‡ (N=797)	PT	150	PRA 11-99%	53/150 (35.3)	NR	NR	NA
Yamauchi J, 1989 (N=28)	DST	19	Crossmatch	6/19 (31.6)	6/6 (100)	0/6 (0)	NA
Albrechtsen D, 1988 (N=701)	RT	476	Crossmatch	NR	NR	NR	NA
Brynger H, 1988 (N=459)	RT	289	Positive PRA	NR	NR	NR	NA
Bucin D, 1988 (N=116)	RT	79	Presence of antibodies	30/79 (38.0)	30/30 (100)	0/30 (0)	NA
Kerman RH, 1988 (N=320)	RT	220	Highest PRA	NR	NR	NR	NA
Madrenas J, 1988 (N=287)	RT	233	PRA >50%	NR	NR	NR	NA
Takiff H, 1988 (N=NR)	RT	NR	Current, peak PRA	NR	NR	NR	NA
Alarif L, 1987 (N=126)	RT	126	PRA ≥ 10 %	16/126 (12.7)	16/16 (100)	0/16 (0)	NA
Garcia VD, 1987 (N=104)	DST	35	T-warm or B-warm donor specific crossmatches	NR (29.8)	NR	NR	NA
Ho-Hsieh H, 1987 (N=51)	RT	33	NR	NR	NR	NR	NA

Study, Year (N=)	Type of transfusion	Number of transfused patients ($N_T=$)	Assessment	Number of transfused patients who were sensitized N_s/N_T (%)	Number of sensitized patients who were transplanted with planned kidney n/N_s (%)	Number of sensitized patients who were not transplanted with planned kidney n/N_s (%)	Comments
Melzer JS, 1987 (N=212)	RT	163	Peak PRA >50%	12/163 (7.4)	12/12 (100)	0/12 (0)	NA
Salvatierra O, 1987 b[§]	DST	302	A positive T warm crossmatch or a positive B warm crossmatch with a concomitant positive fluorescence-activated cell sorter crossmatch	NR	NR	NR	NR
CMTSG, 1986 (N=291)	RT	44	Current cytotoxic antibody > 10% Highest cytotoxic antibody > 50%	NR	NR	NR	NA
Norman DJ, 1986 (N=43)	RT	25	Crossmatch	NR	NR	NR	NA
Sanfilippo F, 1986 (N=3,628)	RT	NR	Peak and current PRA levels	NR	NR	NR	NA
Sabbaga E, 1985 (N=40)	DST	20	Crossmatch	NR	NR	NR	NA
Sanfilippo F, 1985 (N=107)	LP PRC Mixed	45 42 20	PRA ≥ 20%	NR NR NR	NR NR NR	NR NR NR	NA NA NA
d'Apice AJ, 1984 (N=337)	RT	281	Presensitization: peak reactivity > 25% of panel	NR	NR	NR	NA

Study, Year (N=)	Type of transfusion	Number of transfused patients (N$_T$=)	Assessment	Number of transfused patients who were sensitized N$_S$/N$_T$ (%)	Number of sensitized patients who were transplanted with planned kidney n/N$_S$ (%)	Number of sensitized patients who were not transplanted with planned kidney n/N$_S$ (%)	Comments
Flechner SM, 1984 (N=36)	RT	21	NR	NR	NR	NR	NA
Guillou PJ, 1984 (N=116)	RT	64	NR	NR	NR	NR	NA
Jeffery JR, 1984 (N=NR)	RT	33	Cytotoxic antibodies	NR	NR	NR	NA
Ting A, 1984 (N=298)	RT	170	NR	NR	NR	NR	NA
Velasco N, 1984 (N=96)	RT	NR	NR	NR	NR	NR	NA
Cheigh JS, 1983 (N=62)	RT	47	Percent lymphocytotoxicity	NR	NR	NR	NA
Cho SI, 1983 (N=178)	RT	159	PRA ≥ 10%	57/159 (35.8)	57/57 (100)	0/57 (0)	Immunization status was retrospectively evaluated in the included patients who had already received transplantation
Garvin PJ, 1983 (N=92)	RT	71	PRA > 10%	NR	NR	NR	NA
Kerman RH, 1983 (N=104)	RT	NR	Crossmatch	NR	NR	NR	NA
Madsen M, 1983 (N=158)	RT	142	Crossmatch	NR	NR	NR	NA

Study, Year (N=)	Type of transfusion	Number of transfused patients (N_T=)	Assessment	Number of transfused patients who were sensitized N_S/N_T (%)	Number of sensitized patients who were transplanted with planned kidney n/Ns (%)	Number of sensitized patients who were not transplanted with planned kidney n/Ns (%)	Comments
Muller GA, 1983 (N=80)	RT	NR	Crossmatch	NR	NR	NR	NA
Myburgh JA, 1983 (N=262)	RT	193	Crossmatch	NR	NR	NR	NA
Okiye SE, 1983 (N=165)	RT	130	Preformed antibodies >5%	NR	NR	NR	NA
Rao KV, 1983 (N=300)	RT	251	Cytotoxic antibodies >50% assessed at time of transplant	NR	NR	NR	NA
Richie RE, 1983 (N=389)	RT	284	NR	NR	NR	NR	NA
Spees EK, 1983 (N=3,042)	RT	2473	Percent reactive antibody: cytotoxicity against a panel	NR	NR	NR	NA
Zeichner WD, 1983 (N=77)	PT	61	Cytotoxic antibody levels >10%: screened against panel	4/59 (6.8)	4/4 (100)	0/4 (0)	Immunization status was retrospectively evaluated in the included patients who had already received transplantation
Betuel H, 1982 (N=246)	PT RT	165 81	Anti-HLA antibodies	67/165 (40.6) 27/81 (33.3)	67/67 (100) 27/27 (100)	0/67 (0) 0/27 (0)	Immunization status was retrospectively evaluated in the included patients who had already received transplantation
Chu D, 1982 (N=32)	RT	22	Pretransplant antibody level; crossmatch	NR	NR	NR	NA
Dewar PJ, 1982 (N=357)	LD: RT CD: RT	77 188	Lymphocytotoxic crossmatch	NR	NR	NR	NA

Study, Year (N=)	Type of transfusion	Number of transfused patients ($N_T=$)	Assessment	Number of transfused patients who were sensitized N_s/N_T (%)	Number of sensitized patients who were transplanted with planned kidney n/Ns (%)	Number of sensitized patients who were not transplanted with planned kidney n/Ns (%)	Comments
Fehman I, 1982 (N=130)	RT	85	Crossmatch	NR	NR	NR	NA
Flechner SM, 1982 (N=100)	RT	89	Preformed antibody >10%: assessed against random panel of lymphocytes; crossmatch	NR	NR	NR	NA
Fradet Y, 1982 (N=121)	RT	93	Lymphocytotoxic antibodies, pre- and post-transplant	NR	NR	NR	NA
Frisk B, 1982 (N=347)	PT RT	116 191	Cytotoxic antibody	NR	NR	NR	NA
Fuller TC, 1982 (N=156)	RT	135	>10% panel alloantibody reactive	42/135 (31.1)	42/42 (100)	0/42 (0)	All patients received transplant
Glass NR, 1982 (N=94)	RT	45	NR	NR	NR	NR	NA
Kovithavongs T, 1982 a|| (N=48)	RT	25	Lymphocyte mediated cytotoxicity assessed	NR	NR	NR	NR
Kovithavongs T, 1982b|| (N=48)	RT	15	Lymphocyte mediated cytotoxicity assessed	4/7 (57.1)	4/4 (100)	0/4 (0)	Immunization status was retrospectively evaluated in the included patients who had already received transplantation
Mendez R, 1982 (N=67)	RT	54	Preformed lymphocytotoxins	18/49 (36.7)	18/18 (100)	0/18 (0)	Preformed lymphocytotoxins was not assessed in 5 transfused and transplanted patients
Sirchia G, 1982 (N=65)	RT	65	Lymphocytotoxic antibodies; crossmatch	NR	NR	NR	NA

E - 9

Study, Year (N=)	Type of transfusion	Number of transfused patients (N_T=)	Assessment	Number of transfused patients who were sensitized N_S/N_T (%)	Number of sensitized patients who were transplanted with planned kidney n/N_S (%)	Number of sensitized patients who were not transplanted with planned kidney n/N_S (%)	Comments
Walker JF, 1982 (N=204)	RT	137	NR	NR	NR	NR	NA
Feduska, 1981a[||] (N=732)	RT	517	Percent of cytotoxic antibodies >10%	32/517 (6.2)	32/32 (100)	0/32 (0)	All patients included in this subgroup received transplantation
Feduska, 1981b[||] (N=977)	RT	666	Percent of cytotoxic antibodies >10%	57/666 (8.6)	35/57 (56.1)	25/25 (100)	All patients in this subgroup were on hemodialysis, and transplantations were not offered
Hurst PE, 1981 (N=168)	RT	109	NR	NR	NR	NR	NA
Persijn GG, 1981 (N=52)	LP/LDP	52	Lymphocytotoxic antibodies: against a panel of 50 antigens; crossmatch	NR	NR	NR	NA
Sirchia G, 1981 (N=484)	RT	325	Presence of lymphocytotoxic antibodies, positive B cell crossmatch	NR	NR	NR	NA
Thorsby E, 1981 (N=129)	RT	73	Crossmatch	NR	NR	NR	NA
Van Es A, 1981 (N=269)	RT	244	NR	NR	NR	NR	NA
Corry RJ, 1980 (N=94)	RT	45	NR	NR	NR	NR	NA
Fehman I, 1980 (N=229)	RT	159	HLA antibodies	28/159 (17.6)	28/28 (100)	0/28 (0)	Immunization status was retrospectively evaluated in the included patients who had already received transplantation

Study, Year (N=)	Type of transfusion	Number of transfused patients (N_T=)	Assessment	Number of transfused patients who were sensitized N_S/N_T (%)	Number of sensitized patients who were transplanted with planned kidney n/Ns (%)	Number of sensitized patients who were not transplanted with planned kidney n/Ns (%)	Comments
Jakobsen A, 1980 (N=301)	RT	157	NR	NR	NR	NR	NA
Spees EK, 1980 (N=995)	RT	829	Current and Peak PRA levels: data provided (0, >0)	427/829 (51.5) [Peak >0]	427/427 (100)	0/427 (0)	Immunization status was retrospectively evaluated in the included patients who had already received transplantation
Andrus C, 1979 (N=55)	RT	NR	Antibody incidence	NR	NR	NR	NA
Fauchet R, 1979 (N=71)	RT	45	HLA presensitization	NR	NR	NR	NA
Hourmant M, 1979 (N=163)	RT	121	NR	NR	NR	NR	NA
Oei LS, 1979 (N=86)#	RT	69	NR	NR	NR	NR	NA
Sengar D, 1979 (N=117)	RT	78	Lymphocytotoxic antibodies	8/78 (10.3)	8/8 (100)	0/8 (0)	Immunization status was retrospectively evaluated in the included patients who had already received transplantation
Werner-Favre C, 1979a** (N=181)	RT	167	Highest level of anti-PBL antibodies	58/167 (34.7) [anti-PBL antibodies ≥5%]	NR	NR	NR
Werner-Favre C, 1979b** (N=101)	RT	87	Highest level of anti-PBL antibodies	19/71 (26.8) [anti-PBL antibodies ≥5%]	19/19 (100)	0/19 (0)	Anti-PBL antibodies results not reported in 16 transfused and transplanted patients
Blamey RW, 1978 (N=32)	RT	10	NR	NR	NR	NR	NA

Study, Year (N=)	Type of transfusion	Number of transfused patients (N_T=)	Assessment	Number of transfused patients who were sensitized N_s/N_T (%)	Number of sensitized patients who were transplanted with planned kidney n/Ns (%)	Number of sensitized patients who were not transplanted with planned kidney n/Ns (%)	Comments
Briggs JD, 1978 a[††]	RT	68	HLA antibodies	NR	NR	NR	NA
Briggs JD, 1978 b[††] (N=159)	RT	63	HLA antibodies	16/63 (25.4)	NR	NR	NA
Jeffrey JR, 1978 (N=44)	RT	20	NR	NR	NR	NR	NA
Jeffery JR, 1978 (N=48)	RT	24	Maximum cytotoxic antibody levels	12/24 (50.0), [max level≥5%]	12/12 (100)	0/12 (0)	Immunization status was retrospectively evaluated in the included patients who had already received transplantation
Stiller CR, 1978 (N=32)	RT	14	NR	NR	NR	NR	NA
Brynger H, 1977 a[‡]	RT	144	HLA-antibodies	NR	NR	NR	Immunization status was retrospectively evaluated in the
Brynger H, 1977 b[‡] (N=244)	RT	42	HLA-antibodies	3/42 (7.1)	3/3 (100)	0/3 (0)	included patients who had already received transplantation
Fuller TC, 1977 (N=90)	RT	80	>20% cytotoxicity with 2 or more cells in panel	16/80 (20.0)	16/16 (100)	0/16 (0)	Immunization status was retrospectively evaluated in the included patients who had already received transplantation
Husberg BO, 1977 (N=95)	RT	65	Lymphocytotoxic antibodies	17/65 (21.5)	17/17 (100)	0/17 (0)	Immunization status was retrospectively evaluated in the included patients who had already received transplantation
Joysey VC, 1977 (N=272)	RT	162	Cytotoxic antibodies	NR	NR	NR	NA
Perkins HA, 1977 (N=126)	RT	99	NR	NR	NR	NR	NA
Persijn GG, 1977 (N=622)	RT	589	Cytotoxic antibodies	NR	NR	NR	NA

Study, Year (N=)	Type of transfusion	Number of transfused patients (N_T=)	Assessment	Number of transfused patients who were sensitized N_s/N_T (%)	Number of sensitized patients who were transplanted with planned kidney n/Ns (%)	Number of sensitized patients who were not transplanted with planned kidney n/Ns (%)	Comments
Polesky HF, 1977 (N=281)	Mixed	248	NR	NR	NR	NR	NA
Sachs JA, 1977 (N=524)	RT	358	Cytotoxic antibodies	NR	NR	NR	NA
Säfwenberg J, 1977 (N=117)	Mixed	65	HLA antibodies	21/63 (33.3)	21/21 (100)	0/21 (0)	Immunization status was retrospectively evaluated in the included patients who had already received transplantation
Walter S, 1977 (N=88)	RT	65	NR	NR	NR	NR	NA
Opelz G, 1974 (N=290)	RT	228	NR	NR	NR	NR	NA
Opelz G, 1973 (N=148)	RT	123	Cytotoxic antibodies	NR	NR	NR	NA
Opelz, 1972 (N= 829)	NR	NR	Cytotoxins	NR	NR	NR	NA

* Results were not reported for the entire transfused population, only for the population who were transfused and transplanted
† Analysis was evaluated using the subgroup population (i.e. Cyclosporine groups)
‡ Pfaff 1989a included nonparous subgroup, and Pfaff 1989b included parous subgroup
§ Salvatierra 1987b included the entire transfused population
‖ Kovithavongs 1982a included patients who received HLA haploidentical transplant, and Kovithavongs 1982b included patients with HLA identical transplant
¶ Feduska 1981a included patients who received deceased donor graft, and Feduska 1981b included patients who were still waiting for transplantation
\# Only results of living donor transplant recipients was included in the analysis, overlapping information with Corry RJ et al, 1980 for the cadaver transplant recipients, and thus not included in this analysis
** Werner-Favre 1979a included the entire study population, and Wener-Favre 1979b included subgroup patients who were screened for anti-PBL antibodies, and were transfused and transplanted.
†† Briggs 1978a included cadaver transplant recipients, and Briggs 1978b included patients receiving hemodialysis.
‡‡ Brynger 1977a included cadaveric renal transplant recipients, and Brynger 1977b included living donor transplant recipients.

Anti-PBL=antiperipheral blood lymphocytes, CD=cadaveric donor transplantation, CMTSG=Canadian Multicenter Transplant Group, DST=donor specific transfusion, HLA=human leukocyte antigen, LD=living donor transplantation, LP=leukocyte-poor transfusions, mPTF=matched pretransplant transfusion, PRC=packed red cell transfusion, PT=protocol transfusion, RT=random transfusion, NA=not applicable, N=Total number of study population, n=number of patients in the subgroup, NR=not reported, NT=Number of transfused patients, Ns=number of sensitized patients,

www.ingramcontent.com/pod-product-compliance
Lightning Source LLC
Chambersburg PA
CBHW081725170526
45167CB00009B/3698